KT-569-758

Care of the Suicidal Person

For Elsevier:

Commissioning Editor: Steven Black
Development Editor: Catherine Jackson
Project Manager: Christine Johnston
Designer: George Ajayi
Illustrations Manager: Merlyn Harvey
Illustrator: David Gardner

Care
of the
Suicidal
Person

John R. Cutcliffe RMN RGN RPN RN BSc(Hons) Nursing PhD

David G. Braithwaite Professor of Nursing, University of Texas (Tyler), USA; Adjunct Professor of Psychiatric Nursing, Stenberg College International School of Nursing; Visiting Professor, University of Ulster, UK; Director, Cutcliffe Consulting

Chris Stevenson RMN BA(Hons) MSc PhD

Chair in Mental Health Nursing, School of Nursing, Dublin College University, Dublin, Ireland; Visiting Professor, University of Ulster, UK

FOREWORDS BY

Ronald Wm. Maris PhD
Distinguished Professor Emeritus, Departments of Psychiatry and Family Medicine, University of South Carolina, Columbia, USA

Paul S. Links MD FRCPC
Arthur Sommer Rotenberg Chair in Suicide Studies, Professor of Psychiatry, Department of Psychiatry, Faculty of Medicine, University of Toronto, Canada

Brian L. Mishara PhD
Director, Centre for Research and Intervention on Suicide and Euthanasia; Professor, Psychology Department, University of Quebec at Montreal, Canada

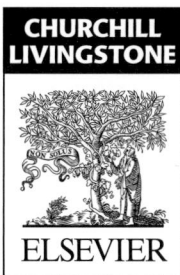

CHURCHILL LIVINGSTONE

ELSEVIER

EDINBURGH LONDON NEW YORK OXFORD
PHILADELPHIA ST LOUIS SYDNEY TORONTO 2007

CHURCHILL
LIVINGSTONE
ELSEVIER

© 2007, Elsevier Limited. All rights reserved.

First published 2007

ISBN-13: 978 0 443 10196 0

British Library Cataloguing in Publication Data
A catalogue record for this book is available from the British Library.

Library of Congress Cataloging in Publication Data
A catalog record for this book is available from the Library of Congress.

Notice
Knowledge and best practice in this field are constantly changing. As new research and experience broaden our knowledge, changes in practice, treatment and drug therapy may become necessary or appropriate. Readers are advised to check the most current information provided (i) on procedures featured or (ii) by the manufacturer of each product to be administered, to verify the recommended dose or formula, the method and duration of administration, and contraindications. It is the responsibility of the practitioner, relying on their own experience and knowledge of the patient, to make diagnoses, to determine dosages and the best treatment for each individual patient, and to take all appropriate safety precautions. To the fullest extent of the law, neither the Publisher nor the Authors assumes any liability for any injury and/or damage to persons or property arising out or related to any use of the material contained in this book.

The Publisher

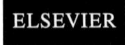
The Publisher's policy is to use **paper manufactured from sustainable forests**

Printed in China

Contents

Chapter 1
Introduction: the Concept of Suicide

Chapter 2
Psychiatric/Mental Health Nursing and Suicide – Policy, Practice and Research

Chapter 3
Research Methods and Suicidology

Chapter 4
Re-connecting the Person with Humanity: the Core Process

Chapter 5
Reflecting an Image of Humanity – Stage One

Chapter 6
Guiding the Individual Back Towards Humanity – Stage Two

Chapter 7
Learning to Live – Stage Three

Chapter 8
Theoretical Refutations and Practice Implications

Foreword

Ronald Wm. Maris

Cutcliffe and Stevenson are on to something absolutely basic to suicide prevention. To oversimplify and slightly banalize what is in fact a sophisticated argument, they see the psychiatric nurse as a 'significant other' for suicidal patients. Their wonderful new book is idiographic, ethnomethodological, qualitative and set in 'grounded theory'.

In Chapter 1 their focus on suicide is multidimensional, multicultural, and developmental. They argue that most suicides have 'suicidal careers' (see Joiner 2005, Maris 1981) over many years and are rooted via social learning, and perhaps genetics, in suicidogenic families of origin as well as in suicidogenic contexts. Their main argument reminds me of Thomas Joiner's recent book (*Why People Die by Suicide*, 2005) in which he suggests that suicides have the 'learned ability to hurt oneself or to enact lethal self-injury'.

Chapter 2 reports that most 'care' by psychiatric/mental health nurses is, unfortunately, mainly direct observation 24/7 for 1 or 2 days. While constant observation may prevent a patient from putting a noose around their neck, it does little or nothing to reduce suicide ideation. In fact such care may paradoxically increase suicidality in the long run. People in hospitals who do observation are often the least skilled, most robotic, custodial, and uninvolved with patients. Thus, observational care may at best only defer, not prevent, suicide. In sum, observation usually is in fact not care. Psychiatrist Alex Pokorny (1983, 1992) reminds us as well that on average suicide assessment identifies about 30% false positives. So, if you had (say) 100 patients on a psychiatric ward, ask yourself if you could even afford to directly observe 30% of them 1:1 24/7 with psychiatric nurses? Obviously not.

Chapter 3 reviews the research design of the book. Cutcliffe and Stevenson's research is qualitative, inductive, and based in what Glaser and Strauss call 'grounded theory'; not in a rigid, formal, preconceived deductive theory of suicide, suicidal behaviour and care. Key concepts of grounded theory are theory generation, theoretical sampling, comparative methods, and theoretical sensitivity. The authors studied intensively 20 former clients who received care for a 'suicidal crisis', especially in South Yorkshire and Newcastle. All interviews were recorded verbatim on audiotapes. Cutcliffe coded the first interviews and then the research team refined the categories and conceptualized interview themes, until the data were 'saturated' and no new themes emerged.

Chapter 4 explains the authors' grounded theory core suicide prevention concept/variable of 'reconnecting the person/patient with humanity'. At first blush this concept sounds vague, abstract, even a little mystical and grandiose; like Jung's notion of the 'collective unconscious'. But what the authors mean here is quite simply and plainly that psychiatric/mental health nurses need to provide intense, warm human contact; a kind of crucial 'transference' (be a 'significant other' to suicidal people) if you will. Suicides are often profoundly 'disconnected' from family and friends. For example, in my survey of Chicago suicides I discovered that 50% of them had zero close friends and were often separated or divorced and living alone.

Note well (my own belief) that 'care' is not the same as 'salvation'. Sometimes we can care and connect with another human being and yet not be able to save them. One also has to query: connected to what? Not all intense connections are beneficent, clearly (see my concept of 'negative interaction' in *Pathways to Suicide*, 1981). Nevertheless, the authors' interviewees' feelings were epitomized by aloneness, isolation, hopelessness, and lack of support or perceived lack of support. All this means in part is that suicidal patients need to be 'touched' in a special way. I am reminded of dying patients asking for pain injections in order to be touched, regardless of what was even in the syringe itself.

Chapter 5 talks about the first phase or stage of 'reflecting an image of humanity'. In this phase there are two key processes or procedures: (1) experiencing intense, warm, care-based human contact, and (2) implicitly (not directly) having the caregiver challenge the patient's suicidal constructs.

This reminds me of Chad Varah and the Samaritans' theme of 'befriending'.

In phase 1 the nurse becomes the emissary or proxy for 'humanity'.

There are some complications with phase 1, I think. For example, what about the well-being of the nurse/caregiver? Or what if the nurse is Nurse Ratched (from *One Flew Over The Cuckoo's Nest*) or Dr Kevorkian? We wonder if unconditional acceptance is always beneficial to the patient (what about 'tough love' for addicts)? Furthermore, interconnectedness is transitive. If so, this phase could make the nurse suicidal and not the suicidal patient more life-affirming.

Undeniably human connections are crucial to well-being. Every time I go to national suicide prevention meetings a close friend of mine from Charleston, South Carolina simply gives me a big HUG (we often say nothing at all). I frequently get more out of that hug than an hour's dry lecture on suicide prevention. Much of Chapter 5 is implicit cognitive behavioural therapy (ala Tim Beck). Remind the patient that constructs are only constructs. Intensify your contacts. Don't watch the clock. Build trust through humour ('If you kill yourself, I'll never talk to you again!').

Chapter 6 explicates Stage 2, in which the nurse guides the individual back to life-affirmation. Through the generous use of interview quotations

from the study subjects the reader sees that this stage includes nurturing insights, strengthening pre-suicidal beliefs, and facilitating a novel, helping relationship. We are told that Stage 2 is not being, but 'doing'. The nurse's relationship with the patient is now at a different pace towards a 'life position.' Both patient and nurse become more aware of the specific type(s) of help needed.

As in Beck's cognitive therapy there is Stage 2 positive reframing of constricted thoughts (such as: 'You know, I have to be miserable or dead.'), removing dysfunctional assumptions ('I am not capable of giving or receiving love.'). In this stage the nurse can reconnect (Query: can one 'reconnect', if you were never connected before?) or redraw on older, pre-illness religious beliefs. One can encourage novel relationships with professionals and not just family and friends (or use professionals to become more open to relationships with family and friends that have atrophied).

Often there will be Stage 2 'Gestalt' or 'Aha!' experiences, where fundamental corrective insights may emerge ('Every time I act like that, I push away the very people I need to sustain me'). The patient has to realize that there is no 'magic pill or magic bullet' that will by itself correct the patient's depression or suicidality. The nurse should teach stress reduction and anxiety management (remember, depression plus anxiety is deadly and often we need to just take the edge off the anxiety).

In Stage 3 (Chapter 7) the patient learns or relearns to live. This may involve re-engaging with their family and friends, not just with their nurse. The nurse needs to deal with existential angst (see my 1982 paper on 'rational suicide') and not superficially dismiss suicidality or thoughts of suicide (as the authors remind us on the very first page of their book, Camus thought that whether or not to suicide was the first and most basic question of philosophy. It's a serious question; not trivial).

The patient needs to reflect: 'Maybe some good could come from all this?' The patient in Stage 3 re-engages in ordinary life. Sylvia Plath (in *The Bell Jar*) says when she emerged from her suicidal depression, it was like a large bell jar was lifted from her body and she could feel the breeze again around her ankles. Hope re-emerges in Stage 3. 'I was sick, but now I am not so sick anymore.' The patient needs to get back to everyday routines that were put in abeyance while they were acutely ill (we are always a little ill; see Kierkegaard's *Sickness Unto Death*) . . . to work, sweat, eat, exercise, have sex, travel, smell and taste things. In Stage 3 the patient embraces the hard work of re-investing in life.

In Chapters 8 through 11, the authors reflect on the conceptual, practical, ethical, and larger implications of their research. Chapter 8 starts off with 'conceptual mirrors' to the extant scientific literature, which support Cutcliffe and Stevenson's grounded theory of caring for the suicidal person. For example, there is interesting and disturbing discharge data, which indicates the highest risk of suicide occurs just after the relationship with the nursing care is terminated or changed at discharge.

Some of the practice implications of the authors' research are: (1) the nurse needs to be comfortable with death and death-talk themselves (research shows that many people go into nursing or medicine because they themselves are uncomfortable with death and dying), (2) talk in order to listen (see Kubler-Ross), (3) training of nurses needs to be more care-focused and less assessment-focused, (4) engage your patients, don't just 'observe' them, (5) move away from the medication-based treatment, being forced on us by managed care, (6) go from suicide risk assessment to suicidal patient care, and (7) adopt a recovery, not cure, model ('There is no cure for life; as long as we are alive, we will have problems').

I wrote a major book on suicide risk assessment (1992) and I know full-well that risk assessment itself never saved anyone's life. We already knew and strongly suspected that most people we assessed were suicidal, otherwise we would not be doing it in the first place. The authors remind us that psychiatric/mental health nurses and their training pay woefully little attention to what nurses might do after risk assessment is completed. Now what? Recovery takes longer than risk-reduction. You are not 'well' just because your GAF score goes from 20 to 50.

Chapter 9 considers the research and training implications of the authors' work. Some of these are: (1) the extent of formal education and training for nurses treating suicidal people, (2) the degree of competence and confidence of the clinical staff, (3) the need for 'action' research (such as the early diagnosis and treatment of depressive disorders), (4) replications of the study's findings in peripheral sites or other countries, and (5) longitudinal comparisons of standard practice groups with psychiatric/mental health nurses with 'care-based' training. Two of the many policy implications of the book's results are (1) that solutions to problems of suicidal people are not in the hands of psychiatrists, but rather in the hands of the patients themselves, and (2) there is a need for more clinical supervision for nurses that care for suicidal persons.

Chapter 10 considers ethical issues in the care of suicidal persons' such as: (1) whom does your body and life belong to?, (2) can suicide ever be 'rational' (or is 'rational suicide' an oxymoron)?, or (3) should nurses ever assist a suicide? Answers to questions like these often turn on moralist, libertarian, or relativist theory perspectives. The chapter suggests that there are interesting parallels to suicide in the bodily risks taken in extreme sports.

For example, do mountain climbers, race car drivers, white-water rafters, sport parachutists, etc., have the right to risk their death in the name of sport?

Cutcliffe and Stevenson point out that much of traditional care of suicidal people is 'paternalistic'. Courts, physicians, nurses often treat patients like children, with few, if any, rights or privileges. The conditions of rational suicide listed by Speijer and Diekstra are discussed (Speijer, a leading Dutch suicidologist, killed himself but before doing so, wrote Diekstra a letter saying his suicide was 'rational' and followed conditions that the two of them had specified earlier). The chapter also reviews case law on suicide. It concludes with the claim that not everyone who suicides is mentally ill, but probably most suicides are irrational in the sense that the perpetrator was often unable to consider his/her best alternative to suicide.

The final chapter, Chapter 11 (written with Frank Campbell), appropriately discusses the huge contribution that suicide survivors make to the care and understanding of suicidal people. This concluding chapter reviews some of the history of the survivor movement. It maintains that suicide bereavement is in many ways dissimilar to standard non-suicidal bereavement. For example, there is more prominent guilt and blame involved in suicidal deaths.

The research of the American Foundation for Suicide Research and the NIMH workshop on survivors in 2003 is reviewed. Among the topics considered are: (1) the impact of suicide on families, (2) social adjustment after a suicide, (3) the heightened risks of suicide for survivors themselves, (4) the role of the first-responder, and (5) the concept of the 'wounded helper'. The chapter concludes with a consideration of how to move from anguish to action and refers the reader to the Baton Rouge Crisis Intervention website.

Cutcliffe and Stevenson have written a remarkable book that has its finger on the heart and pulse of suicidal people. It is carefully crafted and immensely readable. The next time you and your significant other are thinking about going out to dinner, stay home, and take the money you saved and buy this book. The suicidal people in your life will thank you.

Years ago I pondered whether or not I would want a philosopher to talk to, if I were ever thinking about killing myself. 'Duh, no!' Suicide is not so much about thinking clearly or making a rational choice. It's about having the will and ability to keep on living. Life is hard. We need someone or something other than ourselves to live for and we often need help to keep going or to want to keep going.

The lucky among us almost never ever get suicidal. We may find the very idea of suicide bizarre and alien. Our mom and dad, brothers and sisters, lovers, children, friends, and mentors make life do-able and worthwhile or not. Pain, depression, loss, failure, death of others, shame, illness, reversals threaten to undo us all from time to time. The kind of nursing care that Cutcliffe and Stevenson champion in *Care of the Suicidal Person* can help us to invest and reinvest in life, heal us, empower us to keep struggling. Death is nothing. Life is all there is.

Ronald Wm. Maris PhD
Distinguished Professor Emeritus,
Departments of Psychiatry & Family Medicine,
University of South Carolina,
Columbia

Foreword

Paul S. Links

Reading *Care of the Suicidal Person* during a long cross-country flight was as jolting as the landing of the aircraft finally coming back to earth. The 'jolt' or 'grab' of this important book, for me, revolves around three crucial issues.

First, the authors, themselves, describe the barrenness of thought that has been applied to our understanding of the nursing care of the suicidal patient. As a clinician and psychiatrist, I have ordered one-to-one nursing care for many acutely suicidal patients; much as one would request valet parking. Please just return my patient 'in one piece'. Drs Cutcliffe and Stevenson bring their qualitative expertise to understanding the question of how nursing care moves suicidal patients from seeking death to the 'land of the living'. The researchers used modified Grounded Theory and completed in-depth interviews with twenty people who had received formal mental health care for a suicidal crisis after making a serious attempt on their life. Their theory captures how the Psychiatric/Mental Health (P/MH) nurse 'is the bridge that helps the suicidal person re-connect with humanity' (page 51). The authors discuss the core concept of connectedness as being central to the care of the suicidal person and then elaborate their three-stage process of healing that results from the interpersonal presence and professional care of the P/MH nurse.

Second, the proposed theory has a powerful 'grab' with the psychotherapeutic interventions recently proven effective for patients with borderline personality disorder and recurrent suicidal behaviour. The two psychotherapy approaches, Mentalization-Based Treatment (MBT) and Transference Focused Psychotherapy have been proven efficacious in randomized controlled trials in reducing the recurrence of suicidal behavior in these high risk patients. Although, the therapeutic mechanisms for these therapies are still to be proven, the conceptual models resonate closely with the 'feeling disconnected from humanity' that anchors Cutcliffe and Stevenson's theory. For example, MBT proposes to repair the primary deficit in 'mentalization' that results from the patients' experience of insecure attachment to a primary care provider. Fonagy and Bateman (2006) define mentalization as the person's capacity to comprehend and use their knowledge of their own and others' states of mind. The ability to mentalize prevents one from feeling disconnected, isolated and misunderstood. Transference Focused Psychotherapy utilizes the therapeutic relationship to fuse the patient's disconnected internal representations of self and other (Levy et al 2006). Unable to accurately perceive significant others, the person experiences their relationships as isolating and invalidating. I anticipate that this rich theoretical model proposed by Cutcliffe and Stevenson will have a broad influence including enhancing our understanding of the psychotherapies of patients at high risk for suicide.

Finally, this important work should 'jolt' the whole field of suicidology. As the authors note, Edwin Shneidman, the father of suicidology, was committed to studying the individual which led him to his premise of the centrality of 'psychache'. However in the last few decades, the field has been consumed by a search for robust risk factors that would provide certainty in predicting which individuals will die by suicide. I observe that the domination of this quantitative research has only taken us further and further away from the reality of highly suicidal patients. For instance, risk factors, such as the level of hopelessness and suicidal ideation are meaningful predictors about the long term risk for suicide. Yet, these indicators provide only limited understanding of the immediate experience of suicidality. Drs Cutcliffe and Stevenson have shown us the necessity of seeking out the person using qualitative methods in understanding the puzzle of suicide.

Touching on these crucial issues, the reader will anticipate that I strongly recommend this book. All clinicians, psychotherapists, researchers, family members and others concerned with caring for the suicidal person will be enriched by this work.

Paul S. Links MD FRCPC
Arthur Sommer Rotenburg
Chair in Suicide Studies,
Professor of Psychiatry,
Department of Psychiatry,
Faculty of Medicine,
University of Toronto,
Toronto

Foreword

Brian L. Mishara

Suicide attempters and persons who have been hospitalized for psychiatric problems are populations with the highest risks of re-attempting suicide and dying by suicide. Their suicide risk remains high despite the fact that they generally receive hospital treatment in an institutional setting where the staff are aware of the suicide risk and the staff have a clear objective of preventing their potential suicidal behaviours. In this context, one would think that there must be a vast amount of scientific literature about how to treat inpatients in order to reduce their suicide risk. However this is simply not the case. There is a paucity of writings that specifically examine what must occur during a hospital stay in order to reduce the risk of suicidal behaviours. This book addresses this need by providing the first major syntheses of how hospital staff can effectively engage in a therapeutic process with at-risk inpatients in order to reduce their potential of killing themselves.

It is often assumed that when you hospitalize suicidal individuals, the fact that they are in a secure environment and under observation is enough to guarantee some level of protection against self-injurious behaviours. While they are in hospital, suicidal patients may also benefit from medications and possibly psychotherapeutic interventions from a psychiatrist or psychologist. However the reality of the situation is that suicide risk often remains high and most inpatients spend little time receiving treatments. They are left on their own most of the time under the surveillance of nursing staff. The amount of time suicidal patients actually spend interacting with a psychiatrist or other professional is generally minimal, less than an hour a day. In hospital settings, it is the psychiatric or mental health nurses who are the most available to engage in more extensive interactions with suicidal individuals. The nursing staff is also responsible for creating a therapeutic hospital environment to help decrease the suicide risk and prepare the patient for life outside the hospital setting. This book examines the role of the psychiatric or mental health nurse in accomplishing these tasks. Moreover, it examines their role from a perspective that is based upon a sophisticated understanding of contemporary theories of suicidal behaviours as well as extensive clinical experience in working with suicidal inpatients.

Using a grounded theory approach, the authors present analyses of qualitative data to bolster their thesis that there is compelling evidence for the need for a paradigm shift: the traditional role of nurses as observers who assess risk and work to protect is questioned. The material in this book is based upon solid scientific evidence but the application of research findings is continually illustrated with poignant concrete examples. Rather than just reading about what one should be doing or saying or how suicidal patients feel and think, the numerous verbatim quotes help illustrate what to expect in real life situations. This is one of those rare books that is based upon hard science but is also humane and compassionate. The nurse's role is seen as much more than as technicians who go about their tasks of observation and assessment. Rather, the humane dimension of nursing and how nurses should relate to persons under their care is of foremost importance. Suicide prevention is fostered when nursing staff help patients establish a sense of connectedness and when they work to reduce their isolation. This book is essential reading for anyone who works with suicidal individuals in a therapeutic environment. The book illustrates how theories of suicidology and qualitative research can result in specific guidelines for developing therapeutic relationships in institutional settings that hold much promise for preventing suicides.

Brian L. Mishara PhD
Director,
Centre for Research and Intervention on Suicide
and Euthanasia (CRISE),
Professor,
Psychology Department,
University of Quebec, Montreal

Preface

Suicide and acts of suicide are written throughout the tapestry of human history. The tragic truth is that the history of the world is punctuated by suicide and that despite the best efforts of numerous societies, suicide remains a very real contemporary problem. Furthermore, suicide doesn't discriminate. People from all walks of life and from different cultures, and belonging to various social strata have taken their own lives. While the general trend in the Western world (though this cannot be said of all countries) indicates that the risk of suicide increases correspondingly with older age, suicide has been recorded at most points of the life span; indeed recent epidemiological evidence indicates alarmingly rising rates of suicide in 'young men' in many countries. Women, while having lower rates of suicide than men in most countries, are not spared from the risk of one day completing suicide. In actual fact, in some countries that hitherto had relatively low rates of suicide, women now have higher rates than men.

Since Plato's writings, suicide has remained a source of unease and controversy, though it would be inaccurate to posit attitudes towards suicide through the years as constant. Suicide has been viewed differently throughout history, from the different perspectives offered up by the orthodoxies of the time. However, there is one conclusion that has remained inescapable: suicide is acted and played out in human dramas; suicide it seems is inextricably bound up with the experience of the human condition. In order to underscore the ubiquitous nature of suicide, we wish to illustrate and draw attention to some of the well-known figures who have taken their own lives. Some are well publicized, some less so, each instance being a case in point of the non-discriminatory nature of suicide and evidence of the 'ultimate act' in a human drama.

List of Suicides

- Stuart Adamson, (2001), lead singer, *Big Country*.
- Mark Antony, (30 BC), Roman politician and general.
- Howard Armstrong, (1954), inventor FM radio.
- Isobel Barnett, (1980), British TV personality.
- Bruno Bettelheim, (1990), child psychologist.
- Eva Braun, (1945), mistress and then wife of Adolf Hitler.
- Brutus, (42 BC), Roman politician, assassin of Julius Caesar.
- Boudicca, (60/61), Monarch.
- Capucine, (1990), French actress.
- Cleopatra, (30 BC), Egyptian queen, asp.
- Kurt Cobain, (1994), Lead singer rock group Nirvana.
- Dennis Crosby, (1991), son of Bing Crosby, shotgun.
- Lindsay Crosby, (1989), son of Bing Crosby, shotgun.
- George Armstrong Custer, (1876), American general, probable suicide with pistol.
- Gilles Deleuze, (1995), French philosopher.
- Terence Donovan, (1996), English celebrity photographer.

- George Eastman, (1854–1932), American inventor of Kodak camera. Shot himself.
- Ronald 'Buster' Edwards, (1994), British Great Train robber and flower seller.
- John Ellis, (1932), remorseful hangman.
- Brian Epstein, (1967), *Beatles* manager, likely suicide by pills.
- Justin Fashanu, (1998), British footballer.
- James V Forrestal, (1949), Former U.S. Secretary of Defense who quoted Sophocles in his suicide note.
- Sigmund Freud, (1939), psychoanalyst, morphine overdose.
- Charlotte Perkins Gilman, (1935), American feminist and author (Herland).
- Joseph Goebbels, (1945), German Nazi leader.
- Tony Hancock, (1968), British comedian.
- Hannibal, (182 BC), military commander.
- Ernest Hemingway, (1961), American novelist, shotgun.
- Adolf Hitler, (1945), Nazi Germany's leader. Shot/poisoned himself in his bunker.
- Robert E. Howard, (1936), 'Pulp' writer of Conan the Barbarian. Shot himself in the head on June 11, 1936 after learning his mother was in a permanent coma.
- Michael Hutchence, (1997), Australian lead singer of rock group INXS.
- Wafa Idis, (2002), first Palestinian female suicide bomber.
- Judas Iscariot, (1st century), according to the Bible, betrayed Jesus.
- Dr David Kelly, (2003), British scientist, source of BBC story about the September Dossier concerning the invasion of Iraq and the missing evidence of a 'smoking gun'.
- Sándor Kocsis, (1979), Hungarian football (soccer) player, killed himself in Barcelona after diagnosis of cancer.
- Paul Lafargue, (1911), son-in-law of Karl Marx, communist theorist and author of *The Right to Be Lazy*.
- Carole Landis, (1948), actress.
- Florence Lawrence, (1938), Hollywood's first movie star.
- Primo Levi, (1987), Italian author and Auschwitz survivor.

- Peter Llewelyn-Davies, (1960), UK publisher who as a boy was the inspiration for J M Barrie's Peter Pan.
- Jack London, (1916), US novelist (his doctor believed he had committed suicide by overdose of morphine and atropine, but his widow prevailed on a more senior doctor to ascribe the death to uremia, and had the body quickly cremated before an autopsy could be done).
- Joseph Merrick, (1890), UK celebrity known as the 'Elephant Man'; alleged to have committed suicide by allowing his massive head to obstruct his windpipe.
- Marilyn Monroe, (1926–1962), American actress and sex symbol.
- Captain Lawrence Oates, (1880–1912), Polar explorer.
- Nero, (68 AD), Roman Emporer.
- Johnny O'Keefe, (1978), Australian rock legend known as The Wild One, drug overdose.
- Sylvia Plath, (1963), American poetess, author and essayist.
- Richard Quine, (1989), US film director.
- George Reeves, (1959), actor, played *Superman*.
- Michael Ryan, (1987), mass murderer at Hungerford; shot himself as police closed in on him.
- Bobby Sands, (1981), of the IRA, hunger strike.
- George Sanders, (1972), English actor.
- Seneca the Younger, (65), was ordered to commit suicide by the emperor Nero.
- Del Shannon, (1990), American singer.
- Harold Shipman, (2004), imprisoned British doctor found to have killed 250+ of his patients.
- Elizabeth Siddal, (1862), Pre-Raphaelite icon.
- The Singing Nun, (1985), Belgian singer.
- Socrates, (399 BC), philosopher.
- Screaming Lord Sutch, (1999), UK eccentric singer and politician.
- Hunter S. Thompson, (2005), American author.
- Wolfe Tone, (1798), Irish independence leader.
- Alan Turing, (1954), computer scientist and cryptographer, poisoned apple.
- Vincent van Gogh, (1890), Dutch painter.
- Woodbridge Strong Van Dyke, (1941), American film director.

- Sid Vicious, (1979), bass player of the *Sex Pistols*, not long after allegedly killing his girlfriend.
- Pierre-Charles Villeneuve, (1806), French admiral who lost the Battle of Trafalgar.
- Alan Wilson, (1970), musician, leader of *Canned Heat*.
- Virginia Woolf, (1941), English author, drowning.
- Fred West, (1995), husband of convicted British killer Rosemary West. Hanged himself in prison whilst awaiting trial on the same crimes.
- Kenneth Williams, (1988), camp comedian, UK TV personality and diarist.
- Hong Xiuquan, (1864), Chinese leader of the Taiping Rebellion.
- Xiang Yu, (202 BC), the powerful warlord during Chu-Han contention in China.

http://en.wikipedia.org/wiki/List_of_famous_suicides

In addition to each of these 'famous' suicides, much literature, art, and mythology contains many references to suicide, for example, William Shakespeare's *Romeo and Juliet* and Puccini's opera *Madame Butterfly*. Similarly, in the late 18th century, the German author Goethe's *Die Leiden des jungen Werthers*, (which translate to *The Sorrows of Young Werther*), depicts the romantic story of a young man who kills himself because his love proves unattainable. Indeed, a study of suicide in literature was written by the poet Al Alvarez, entitled *The Savage God*.

Accordingly, it can be seen that suicide is a part of human history, it is entrenched in our literature and various cultures, and for the mental health practitioner, it is part of our everyday lives. Yet, while the international academe has made significant advances in the understanding of suicide, it retains a sense of mystery. There are still wide gaps

in our extant literature and, perhaps more worryingly (for the authors anyway), the P/MH nursing care of the suicidal person is not an area of care that can claim to be grounded on an abundance of empirical literature. As a result P/MH nurses have to 'feel their way in the dark' so to speak, and this is an altogether unsatisfactory situation. We hope that in some small way this book may address this theoretical void and equip P/MH nurses with some empirically derived theory to inform their practice.

In the interests of knowledge dissemination, there have been five presentations of the findings that form the basis for this book.

- The first presentation was at the University of North British Columbia, Canada.
- The second at The Postgraduate Institute of Health Care at University of Teesside, United Kingdom.
- The third presentation was at the formal Department of Health dissemination conference day, Exhibition Centre, Doncaster, 21st October 2003.
- The fourth presentation was at the 37th Annual American Association of Suicidology Conference, Miami, USA, April 14th–17th, 2004.
- And the fifth presentation was contained within Professor Chris Stevenson's inaugural professorial lecture at Dublin City University, Ireland, 2005.

All five presentations have been well received (according to the feedback we have heard), and generated many questions from both academic and practice-based staff; perhaps indicating that the implications of the research are far reaching. In each case the presenters were asked, 'When will this study be published?'

Also, according to Professor Ron Maris (1997), few suicidologists have undertaken federally (nationally) funded, original research which is then written into a book (as opposed to journal papers). Thus, it is perhaps worthy of note that the findings contained in this book are reported from one such nationally funded UK study. Accordingly, the authors are delighted to be able to offer this book in response to the needs and requests of practitioners, and partly in response to a 'call' made by one of the leading international authorities on suicide. One final note; how we each individually think of and 'frame' suicide, how we try and understand it and thus the concomitant methodologies we, as an academe of suicidologists, utilize to study suicide, ultimately influence how we try and deal with it. The authors believe that when uncertainty exists, such as in how best to provide care for suicidal people, having a range of conceptualizations rather than forcing premature, fixed *apriori* frameworks, creates more opportunities for effective caring. In the immensely complex human drama that is suicide, it seems unlikely that 'one size will fit all'.

John R. Cutcliffe
and
Chris Stevenson

Contributor

Frank Campbell PhD LCSW CT
Executive Director of the Baton Rouge Crisis Intervention Center, Inc. and the Crisis Center Foundation

Acknowledgements

This book is dedicated to the research participants who gave so willingly of their time, their stories and experiences; without each of you and your willingness to give to others, this research and book would not be.

We would also like to dedicate this book to Professor Edwin Shneidman and Professor Ron Maris whose undoubted contributions to the suicidology academe are required reading for anyone seriously interested in studying suicide.

Our thanks and congratulations to each member of the original research team, Sue Jackson, Paul Smith and by no means least, Professor Phil Barker.

And lastly, we would like to offer our most sincere thanks to Susan Barnes, and the Department of Health Executive, Trent, who funded the original study in the United Kingdom.

Chapter 1

Introduction: the Concept of Suicide

'There is but one philosophical problem, and that is suicide. Judging whether life is or is not worth living amounts to answering the fundamental question of philosophy.'
Camus 1945

CHAPTER CONTENTS

INTRODUCTION

It seems fitting and proper to start a book on suicide with one of the most famous quotations arising out of the 20th century. These words of the existential philosopher Albert Camus are indelibly etched into the vernacular of the contemporary suicidologist; and at the same time, they are not limited or exclusive to the suicidology academe; the concept of suicide is a world-wide phenomenon. Despite this commonality, as with other concepts related to death and dying, suicide remains a mystifying and enigmatic phenomenon. While having this quality of inscrutability, suicide, as Maris et al (2000) point out, has a riveting compulsion to it. Camus' words unequivocally remind us that suicide (and the resultant study of suicide) is one of the most compelling questions facing humankind. For anyone concerned with or involved in the care of suicidal people this philosophical question will resonate most clearly; and here we fully embrace the widest possible encapsulation of people involved in 'care' of the suicidal person – from crisis to helpline workers, survivors of suicide and front-line mental health professionals. Paradoxically, however, given the ubiquity of suicide, and the established academe of suicidologists, one might be forgiven for assuming that a universally accepted definition would exist. Yet this is not the case (Maris et al 2000, Shneidman 1985).

As a result, this chapter begins by examining some of the current definitions of suicide, while recognizing the context that no current universally accepted definition exists. In so doing, the authors accept Shneidman's (1985) and Leenaars' (2004) position that these definitions serve as mnemonics. In other words, they serve as an *aide-mèmoire*, and perhaps offer a starting point for the subsequent discourse around care of the suicidal person. Following this, the chapter looks at the epidemiology of suicide. The chapter offers only an overview or broad 'brush strokes' of international epidemiological data, before focusing in more detail on two countries: Canada and the United Kingdom; for more detailed analyses of these relationships we refer the reader to part two of the excellent *Comprehensive Textbook of Suicidology* (Maris et al 2000) and to David Lester's fine work in this area (see Lester 1992, for example). The chapter then focuses on cultural aspects of suicide before concentrating on examining the tenets of the major theoretical explanations of suicide. This is then followed by a brief examination of additional perceptions of suicide and these are highlighted by drawing on historical and contemporary cases. In drawing this introductory chapter to a close, we reiterate the central tenets that form our contemporary theoretical understanding of suicide and thus the context for caring for the suicidal person.

CONCERNING DEFINITIONS

When does a suicide become a suicide and not one of the other three possible modes (or causes) of death: natural, accidental and homicidal? According to Silverman (1997, p 12): 'after more than 25 years of discussion and debate, there does not exist a universally accepted set of definitions and classifications of suicidal behaviours for the reliable labeling, counting and study of individuals who are at risk for self-destructive injuries'.

Perhaps as an attempt to remedy this situation, the International Academy for Suicide Research formed a task force to attempt to produce a clear understanding (including definitions) of what suicide is, and is not (Leenaars et al 1997). A summary of the key elements of their findings follows:

- Suicide has different definitions depending on the purpose of the definition (e.g. medical, legal, administrative, personal).
- Even classification of suicide within the four WHO modes of death is problematic; it reduces the person down (in a Cartesian way) and thus fails to take account of individual motivations, intentions and more.
- Clustering of suicidal ideation with suicidal acts is also problematic and causes confusion – in that ideas are separate from actions.
- Suicidal acts should be operationally defined; such definitions should include clear descriptions of methods and medical lethality.
- Such definitions should include a definition of circumstances (whether or not the person was alone at the time and whether or not they were likely to remain so until the methods had ceased to have an effect).
- Definition of medical lethality (the degree to which the methods cause or are sufficient to cause death).
- Definition of intent – defined as to have suicide or deliberate self-killing as one's purpose.

Shneidman's undeniable seminal contribution to the suicidology academe includes movement towards a definition (or definitions). In 1973, he suggested that suicide is the human act of self-inflicted, self-intentioned cessation. More latterly, in 1985, Shneidman defined suicide as: 'currently in the western world, suicide is a conscious act of self-annihilation, best understood as a multi-dimensional malaise in a needful individual who defines an issue for which suicide is the best solution' (Shneidman 1985, p 203).

Maris (1981) offers a similar yet more succinct definition wherein he declares that suicide is intentional self-murder. More recently, together with colleagues, Maris et al (2000) offer a very useful analysis of the four elements that *must* be present in order for an act to be constituted as suicide. These are as follows:

- A death must have occurred.
- The death (and thus suicide) must be intended; suicide is not unintentional.
- Suicide is done by oneself and to oneself (although, the current discourse around physician- (practitioner)-assisted suicide might have a bearing on this element of the definition).
- Suicide can be indirect or passive.

While, for some, this search for a concise definition may be regarded as little more than semantics, for others, indeed, many in the suicidology academe, this is a critical and hitherto incompletely answered question. All our research activity, and similarly, our clinical practice, is prefaced by some conceptualization (and therein definition) of suicide. It is worth wondering how, without an accepted conceptualization of the phenomenon, can we as an academe be sure that we are examining the same phenomenon? In the absence of, as many authors have previously written, a standard nomenclature, are we starting from the same point (Rudd 2000, Silverman 1997)? Without this, can we as clinicians know that we are assessing risk of the same phenomenon? These are questions that have bedeviled many a research study on suicide, and the absence of a definition (and associated classification) leads Silverman (1997, p 13) to assert: 'a nomenclature and classification are needed so that we can proceed with studies that accurately correlate psychological states, economic situations, familial factors, environmental conditions, sociological perspectives, biological variables, genetic predisposition, and psychiatric conditions with suicidal ideation, intent, plans and behaviours'.

THE EPIDEMIOLOGY OF SUICIDE: AN OVERVIEW

While it is prudent to acknowledge problems of definition and conceptualization, a great deal of effort, attention, money and human resources have been directed towards determining the epidemiology of suicide. However, even the most ardent supporter of the epidemiological study of suicide would acknowledge two principal obstacles. One: we cannot ignore the somewhat obvious methodological limitation, that being, to borrow research parlance, the 'subjects' themselves cannot be accessed; they are, after all, dead. Thus, we can only ever estimate, albeit with a degree of empirical confidence. Two: all of our best intelligence *apropro* suicide continues to indicate that suicide is relatively rare. Additional methodological problems include the alleged (and mostly accepted view) that many suicides do not get reported and recorded as suicides, resulting in a gross underestimations of actual rates. Various reasons for this under-reporting have been purported, including the difficulty in defining when a suicide is a suicide, the reluctance of some cultures/nations to report suicides (see Chap 10 for more detail of this), and the stigma that still, for some, is associated with suicide.

Nevertheless, there appears to be a reasonable degree of consensus within the suicidology community that official statistics of suicide can be used to produce reasonably accurate findings and that international comparisons can produce useful and illuminating results. Recent data retrieved from the World Health Organization (2002) indicates the global rate of suicide for countries that had data available, and these are included in Figure 1.1.

It is perhaps startling to realize that, according to the World Health Organization (2002), approximately one million people died as a result of suicide in the year 2000. This translates to 16 people per 100 000 population having taken their own life; that is one death every 40 seconds! Consequently, one can assert with a significant degree of empirical confidence that suicide is a global problem. Perhaps more worryingly, this problem is growing. Despite a substantial research effort and the production of an associated literature, suicide rates continue to rise in many countries. The persuasive evidence provided by the WHO (2002) indicates that the global rate of suicide has continued to rise since 1950. In 1950 the global suicide rate for men was 16 per 100 000 and the rate for women was 5 per 100 000, whereas in 1995, the global suicide rate for men was 25 per 100 000, and the rate for women was 7 per 100 000. The WHO (2002) statistics illustrate how, during the last 45 years, suicide rates have increased by 60% world-wide to

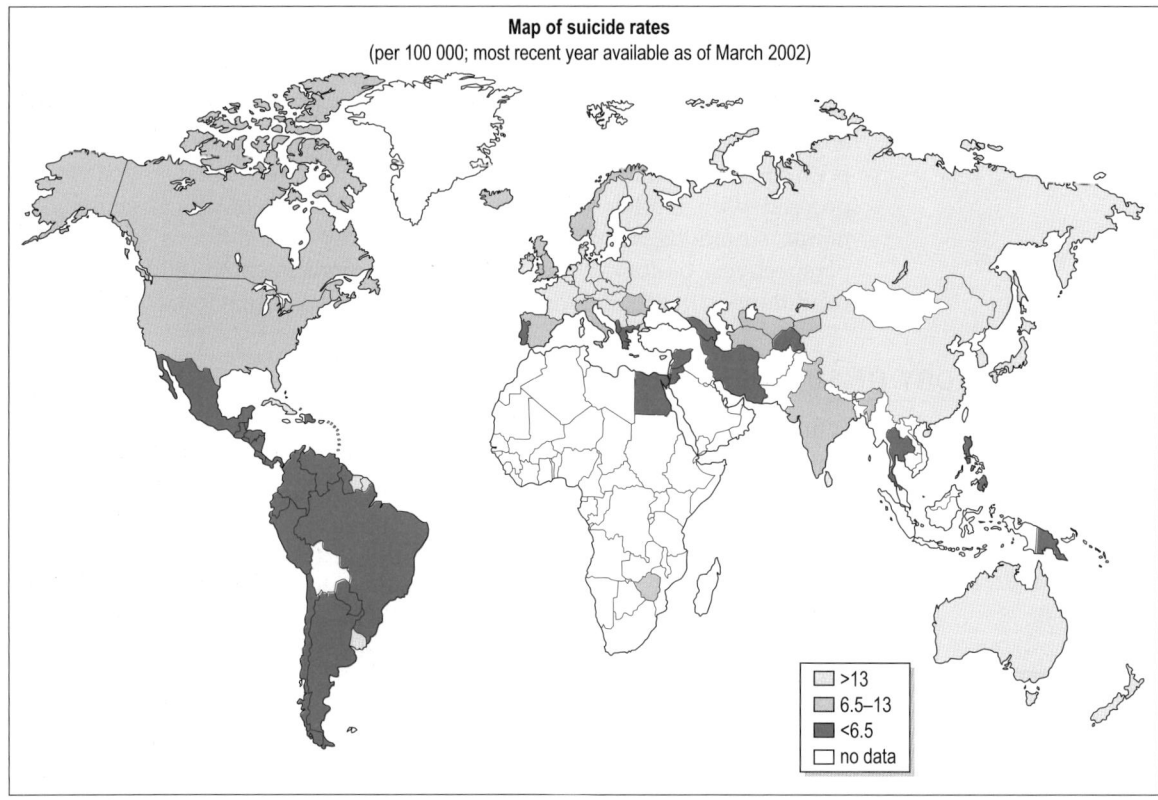

Figure 1.1 World Health Organization data on 2002 global suicide rates. Suicide rates and absolute numbers of suicides by country. Reproduced from the World Health Organization website, with permission.

the extent that suicide is now one of the three 'leading' causes of death among those aged 15–44 years (for both sexes). Perhaps even more alarming is the World Health Organization's (2002) evidence which indicates that attempted suicide is 20 times more common than completed suicide. While the WHO acknowledges that suicide is often associated (and linked to) mental health disorders, it is heartening to see that the WHO recognizes that suicide results from many complex sociocultural factors and appears to be more likely to occur during particular periods of socioeconomic, family and individual stressful times (e.g. loss of a loved one, loss of employment, loss of honour).

Canadian and United Kingdom epidemiology of suicide

Given the affiliations of the authors at the time of undertaking the study focused on in this book, we have chosen to include some epidemiological data from Canada and the United Kingdom in an attempt to illustrate: the types of studies that are undertaken, trends in some 'western' countries, difficulties in establishing accurate data, and the identification of certain high-risk groups.

Canada

According to WHO data and the Canadian Association for Suicide Prevention (2004) Canadian National Suicide Prevention Strategy, the suicide rate in Canada is in the top third of those countries reporting data to the WHO. More worryingly, the suicide rate for Canadian youth is the third highest in the industrialized world. Since 1950, the rate of suicide has risen by 122%. This translates to approximately 10 Canadians killing themselves each day; it accounts for 2% of all Canadian deaths and it is the leading cause of death for Canadian males aged between 10 and 49. Perhaps not surprisingly, many Canadian epidemiological focused studies have attempted to determine the prevalence and distribution of suicide. According to the Canadian Institute for Health Research's (CIHR)/Health Canada (White 2003) descriptive summary of Canadian suicide research, there have been approximately 50 such studies. National level studies have been undertaken to determine overall trends (Beneteau 1988, Lester 1988, 2000, Mao et al 1990, Reed et al 1985). Recent 'overall' national data (Centre for Suicide Prevention 2005) indicate that in 2001, 3692 Canadians died by suicide or from injuries resulting from intentional self-harm. Of these, 2870 were males and 822 were females. This translates to a standard mortality rate of 11.9 per 100 000 of the population. More worrying, the rate for males was 18.6 and the rate for females was 5.2 per 100 000. The highest rates were recorded in the age group 45–49 (males and females combined). It should be noted that the Centre for Suicide Prevention (2005) points out that these data should be considered with a degree of caution, particularly given that no official registry collects data on suicide in Canada. More recently, the long awaited (and most welcome) 'Blueprint for a Canadian National Suicide Prevention Strategy' (Canadian Association for Suicide Prevention (2004)) noted that over 4000 Canadians die by suicide each year and many more, perhaps 100 times as many, deliberately harm themselves. Further, in 1998–1999, 22 887 hospital discharges for suicide attempts or intentional self-inflicted injury were recorded (Canadian Association for Suicide Prevention (Blueprint) 2004).

In addition to these broad, overall studies, the CIHR/Health Canada (White 2003) descriptive summary of Canadian suicide research points out that much work has focused on the prevalence of suicide associated with specific 'variables'. For example:

- Age, gender, geographic region (Dyck et al 1988, Hutchcroft & Tanney 1989).
- Country-of-origin (Strachan et al 1990).
- Birth rates (Lester 2000).
- Socio-demographic factors (Hasselback et al 1991).

The CIHR/Health Canada's (White 2003) descriptive summary document also provides an overview of certain trends in more detail by focusing in on smaller geographical areas (i.e. within certain provinces and/or regions) (Barnes et al 1986, Caron et al 1995, Chiefetz et al 1987, Issacs et al 1998, Lester 1995). Still more work has occurred that has focused on specific social factors and suicide, such as:

- Ethnicity, immigration status (Trovato 1986).
- Marital status (Trovato 1991).

- Social and economic correlates of suicide (Leenaars et al 1993, Leenaars & Lester 1988, 1995).
- Gender in adolescents (Pinhas et al 2002).
- Attitudes towards suicide (Bagley & Ramsey 1989) and cross cultural comparisons (Canada and the United States) (Leenaars & Lester 1994).

As with other countries and associated suicidology scholars, Canadian researchers have undertaken studies to identify certain 'high-risk' groups or populations. Some of these groups/populations have similarly been identified in many other nations, suggesting a degree of commonality and transferability (e.g. people with mental health problems also found to be a high-risk group in UK, USA, Ireland, Finland, Norway, and aboriginal populations in Australia, New Zealand and the USA.) The CIHR/Health Canada (White 2003) descriptive summary document highlights the following high-risk groups and associated Canadian researchers:

- Young people (de Man et al 1992, Kidd 2001, Kidd & Kral 2002).
- Older adults (also known as 'the elderly') (Duckworth & McBride 1996, Marion et al 1999, Mireault & de Man 1996, Quan et al 2002).
- Aboriginal populations (Bagley 1991, Chandler & Lalonde 1992, Lester 1996, Kirmayer et al 1998, Kral et al 2000, Lester 1996, Sigurdson et al 1994).

United Kingdom

According to the data contained in the latest summary issued by the UK Department of Health (2005), published in the 2nd Annual Report from the National Suicide Prevention Strategy for England, the suicide rate in the United Kingdom has dropped slightly. In 1995–1997, the suicide rate per 100 000 population was 9.2, whereas the figure for 2001–2003 was 8.6 per 100 000. According to the report, this indicates a drop of 6% from the baseline rate. Nevertheless, this indicates approximately, 5198 suicide deaths each year in the United Kingdom and this translates to approximately 14.25 people in the UK killing themselves each day. Earlier data (Charlton et al 1994a, b) show that, between the years 1946 and 1990 in the United Kingdom, the rates for younger males (45 and under) had risen markedly, whereas the rates for older males have steadily declined. This trend has continued to the extent that, according to the Department of Health (2005) report, younger males now have a higher rate than older males.

The male/female variation found in Canadian epidemiological studies is echoed in the UK where a ratio of male/female completed suicide is recorded at just over 3:1. This difference is most marked in the 'young' category (25–34 age group), and it declines steadily as age increases until over 50, where it stablizes at about 2.5:1.

In terms of international comparisons, and these data should be treated with a degree of caution due to differences in reporting and recording, the United Kingdom is in the lower third (Kerkhof & Kunst 1994). Indeed, the UK fairs favourably in comparison to other European countries. However, as with other European countries, certain parts of the UK (e.g. Scotland) have a distinctly higher rate and, further, rates vary across regions within countries.

As with Canadian studies, many UK epidemiological focused studies have attempted to determine the prevalence and distribution of suicide. National level studies have been and continue to be undertaken to determine overall trends (Charlton et al 1994a, b, Department of Health 2001, 2005).

In addition, to these broad, overall studies, as within Canada, much work has focused on the prevalence of suicide associated with specific 'variables'. For example:

- Age, gender, geographic region (Charlton et al 1992, Kelly & Charlton 1995).
- Suicide rates in certain cities (Hawton & Fagg 1992, Hawton et al 1994, Platt et al 1988).
- Socio-economic factors (and deprivation) (Gunnell et al 1995)

As with Canadian studies, many UK epidemiological focused studies have attempted to determine the link (if any) between specific social factors and risk of suicide, including:

- Employment status (Charlton et al 1987, Crombie 1990, Fox & Shewry 1988, Moser et al 1987).
- Marital status (Charlton et al 1994b).

As with other countries and associated suicidology scholars, UK epidemiologists and researchers have undertaken studies to identify certain 'high-risk' groups or populations, such as:

- People with mental health problems (Barraclough et al 1974, Hawton 1987, Powell et al 2000).
- Prison populations (Department of Health 2001, 2005, Dooley 1990, Lloyd 1990).
- People with substance use/misuse problems (Hawton et al 1989, Pierce-James 1967).

While these and other epidemiological data should be treated with caution, several interesting themes or trends appear to be evident in these data, including:

1. Suicide remains a major, global health problem.
2. Suicide rates are not consistent over time in some countries, yet they remain fairly stable in other countries.
3. Suicide rates vary according to gender, with males most commonly showing a significantly higher risk, although this is not always the case: see recent data from China where females have a higher recorded rate than males (Phillips et al 1999).
4. Age is an important demographic variable, with Western countries showing a discernable trend of risk of suicide generally increasing with age, although the rise in rates of suicide in young males in many of these countries is perhaps the most alarming epidemiological trend of late.
5. High-risk groups do appear to exist, although these are far from consistent across different countries.
6. One commonality across many countries is that suicide rates have a very high or marked regional variation.

7. However, one cannot necessarily extrapolate from the rates of one country to another.
8. Despite our best efforts at understanding and preventing suicide over the last 50 years, it is fair to say that our efforts have met with (at best) only limited (and perhaps isolated pockets) of success.

THEORETICAL PERSPECTIVES OF SUICIDE: AN OVERVIEW

Irrespective of the particular stance that one adopts to view suicide, one inevitably either adopts, forms, or modifies a theoretical perspective of suicide. All formal areas of study, including suicidology, have a number of core concepts that pertain to their field of enquiry. For example, some of the concepts of importance to suicidologists include: lethality, motive and intent, methods, hopelessness, constricted thoughts and rational suicide. Theories of suicide have been present since the formal beginnings of the study of suicide, and perhaps commenced their theorizing by noting phenomena (e.g. Durkheim noted that the stronger the integration of the religious community, the greater its preservative value on the individual: and he termed this – a coefficient of preservation). Suicidologists who are interested in developing their knowledge base then appear to be attuned to the phenomena around them. According to Meleis (1985), there are two stages in this process. The first stage is 'Attention Grabbing'. Here some clinical situation, event, cultural nuance, behaviour or activity attracts one's attention and he or she develops a hunch about it. This may occur concurrently or retrospectively. This is followed by a more deliberate 'Attention Giving' stage where the suicidologist asks questions such as:

- What has attracted my attention?
- When does it occur?
- Why does it happen?
- Does it have a function?
- Can I describe it?
- Is it similar or different from other happenings?
- It is related to time or place?
- Under what conditions do I observe it, hear it, touch it?
- Does it vary? Under what circumstances?

(From Cutcliffe & McKenna 2004)

As a result, a number of theories of suicide have been purported, each of which contain a number of concepts (and definitions), propositions, laws (conditions under which the propositions hold 'true') and an examination of these will help the reader to understand suicide. Importantly, it is crucial to point out that, given the multi-dimensional nature of suicide, what appear to be (at first glance) conflicting theories can paradoxically add to our more complete understanding rather than leave us at an impasse. One does not necessarily have to consider theories of suicide in the Aristotelian 'either – or' paradigm; it is more accurate and, the authors would argue, more in keeping with the complexity of suicide, to consider it more in terms of a 'post-modernist' 'both – and' view.

Biological theories

It is inescapable that humans are, at least in part, biological beings. However, reducing the explanation of suicide down to a simple causal relationship between neurochemicals (most often serotonin, dopamine and the hypothalamic–pituitary–adrenal (HPA) axis) would appear to be a counterproductive stance. For that matter, the slavish adherence to one theory as having full explanatory potential, irrespective of the particular theoretical view, would be similarly restrictive. It should be acknowledged that, since the seminal study of Asberg et al (1976), in which they reported a relationship between suicidal behaviour and low levels of cerebrospinal fluid 5-hydroxyindoleacetic acid (5-HIAA – the principal metabolite of serotonin) in depressed patients, a number of studies have been undertaken in this area. Some of these have added to this body of knowledge. Interestingly, a former president of the AAS, Dr Drew Slaby (1994), notes additional research undertaken by Asberg et al (1990) which found similar decreases in CSF levels of 5-HIAA in *healthy* individuals. As with many other suicide studies, post-mortem studies are bedeviled with methodological limitations; not least the possibility of post-mortem delay. The eminent British suicidologist Dr Keith Hawton, along with van Heeringen (Hawton & van Heeringen 2000), concluded that there is very little secure empirical knowledge regarding the neurobiology of suicide. Nevertheless, the evidence of, in some cases, serotonergic abnormalities in the brains of suicide victims should not be ignored; there is evidence to suggest that decreased serotonergic functioning is associated with suicidal behaviour.

Social and cultural theories

While the focus in suicidology is most often the individual, or on individuals, suicide is inevitably played out in social and cultural contexts; indeed there is a well established body of literature that shows how social and cultural forces figure prominently in the dynamics of suicide (Maris 1997b). Further, even the most cursory examination of the extant literature will illustrate that huge variation in cultural views/conceptualizations of suicide exist. (See the volume *Suicide: Individual, Cultural and International Perspectives* (1997) edited by Leenaars et al for an excellent set of examples of these cultural and international variations.) Berman et al (2005) write that: 'culture is the nutrient medium in which the organism is cultivated'.

Berman et al's comment appears to be insightful and accurate, particularly when one considers some of the evidence of certain cultures having significantly higher rates (when compared to the rates for the general population). For example, Maris et al (2000) draw attention to the stark contrast in suicide rates between certain countries. They highlight how some countries (e.g. Nigeria, Albania) – and the authors of this current text would add the supporting evidence of some populations of certain North American aboriginal bands – have virtually no suicide rates. This is contrasted with other countries (e.g. Hungary, Lithuania, Latvia, Estonia) having extremely high suicide rates. Further, international variations in suicide rate recorded in numerous texts (see, for example, World Health Organization 2002) are difficult to ignore, methodological problems in establishing these national baseline data notwithstanding. As a result, and given the vivid and startling nature of some of these differences, one might safely conclude that culture appears to have an effect on the suicide rate.

From Durkheim's seminal work on suicide, many authors have added to our body of knowledge concerning the effect of culture (or more likely effects), on suicide. Some have even posited the possibility of a *suicidogenic* national character (see Maris et al 2000). Such groups are posited as those who are set apart from others on the basis of key cultural differences (e.g. attitudes, meanings attached to the act, customs, language, etc.) towards or about suicide. This leads to an interesting question, among others, that is: is there something about belonging to one of these national cultural groups that *ipso facto* causes one to be at a higher risk of suicide? While the authors of this book would not wish to suggest that culture does not have a profound effect on suicide, we would like to draw attention to Takahashi's (1997) discerning remarks. He states: 'despite the fact that some cultural differences in suicide admittedly exist in different societies and that these are important, they cannot explain every aspect of suicide'. Further, he continues: 'from my albeit limited knowledge and experience, it appears as that there are more similarities than differences in suicide among various cultures.'

The veracity of such a view may be increased when one examines certain historical and highly contextual views of suicide (see below for details of these, e.g. suicide in the Roman Empire and suicide within the military). One should also acknowledge that while culture clearly does have an influence on suicide, cultures themselves are constructs and are not static entities. Leenaars (2004) draws attention to the example of the Japanese suicide warrior and the North American aboriginal warrior suicide, and how such suicide deaths were historically regarded as glorious, to illustrate the ever changing nature of culture. As a result of considering some of the literature in this area, a number of key points become evident:

- Culture clearly has an effect on the rate of suicide, but cannot in and of itself account for all national variations.
- The possibility of suicidogenic cultures should not be dismissed, although we add a caveat here – namely:
  - It would be unwise and epidemiologically misleading to automatically stereotype certain cultures as high-risk or low-risk, the huge variation in suicide rates among North American native bands being a case in point – thus, perhaps, indicating the existence of certain suicide subcultures?
  - Culture itself appears to have a reciprocal relationship with suicide – with incidences of suicide effecting how suicide is viewed within the culture (at times, possibly normalizing it) and the views of suicide perhaps contributing to the suicide rate.

Psychological theories

A great deal of work has been produced which can be categorized as contributing to the psychological theories of suicide. While recognizing that overlap between individual theories can (and does) exist, the authors have adopted Leenaar's (2004) useful categorization of psychological theories of suicide into the four perspectives of: psychoanalytical, cognitive-behavioural, social learning and multi-dimensional.

Psychoanalytical perspectives

Freud pioneered the psychoanalytical theories of suicide, suggesting that the cause was the loss of a significant object (e.g. a person). The suicidal person, Freud wrote, is identifying with this rejecting (or lost) person; and the identification is based on the highly significant and meaningful emotional attachment. For Freud, suicide is motivated by intentions within the person's unconscious. Even though the suicidal person may be conscious of his/her plan to engage in suicide, this is an unconscious rejection of the significant object. Thus, the anger/hatred felt (unconsciously) towards the object person is then redirected back upon themselves.

Cognitive–behavioural

Unquestionably, Aaron Beck (and colleagues) have made a huge contribution to cognitive-behavioural theories (and approaches to treatment) of suicide. For cognitive behavioural-therapists, suicide is bound up with depression or perhaps, appropriately, with a sense of hopelessness. From their position of hopelessness, suicidal people have a constricted view of the world (and their place in it), and subsequently see suicide as the only plausible solution to their hopeless position. Such people will have unrealistic and pervasive negative views of their future; it cannot improve and is only likely to get worse. These pervasive, negative constricted thoughts are not limited to the world, they also have such negative views of themselves. Self-blame, low self-esteem/worth, self-criticism are all compounded by interpreting events in a negative way. Furthermore, a number of distortions or errors of thought occur (e.g. negative bias, magnification of minor problems, over generalizing, and selective abstraction). Suicide is thus thought of as a relief or escape from the intolerable pain and is thus a more desirable option than the continued struggle of life.

Social learning

The prominent suicidologist Dr David Lester has developed the classic psychological theories of conditioning (Pavlov, Skinner) and synthesized this with Bandura's theory and thus posits that suicide is a learned behaviour. Suicide results from one's childhood experiences and from the forces and factors encountered in the environment. For these theorists, suicide is thus a shaped behaviour; it has been reinforced in the suicidal person's environment and especially through the person's experiences of being reared as a child. Social learning theories of suicide believe the person has learned not to show any outwards signs of aggression and instead must turn this anger inwards upon themselves. Social learning theories posit that suicide can be a manipulative act, and that suicidal people have not been adequately or sufficient socialized into the 'normal' values of life and death. A number of possible factors or phenomena exist that can serve to reinforce the suicide such as, cultural nuances, 'copycat' (modelling) suicide, and suicide in significant others.

Multi-dimensional

Shneidman (1985, 1997) has long and repeatedly advocated the multidimensional view of suicide. In Shneidman's view the key concept is psychache; unbearable or intolerable psychological pain. This pain is pervasive, it occupies all the person's awareness and has no foreseeable end point. This pain inevitably results from unmet and/or unfulfilled needs and this is experienced as a significantly traumatic event. In such situations then, suicide provides the only possible escape from this unbearable and unceasing pain. As such, it is an end to the pain, brought about by the ending of one's consciousness, that is sought by the suicidal person. As with cognitive-behavioural theories, the suicidal person's thoughts are constricted; the pervasive feelings of hopelessness and helplessness lead to a sense of heightened disturbance, what Shneidman terms, perturbation. Accordingly, the suicidal person wishes to get out, to leave, to be elsewhere.

(adapted from Leenaars 2004)

Lifespan theories: suicide pathways or trajectories

A further and immensely useful theoretical view of suicide is that provided by Professor Ron Maris, and there is growing recognition and support within the scientific academe of suicidologists for Maris' idea of a *pathway(s)* or *trajectory(s)* of suicide (Leenaars 1991, Maris 1981, 1990, Shneidman 1997). In this conceptualization, the developmental-existential perspective of suicide is purported. It is predicated as a person's inability or refusal to accept the terms of the human condition (Maris 1981) as the endpoint of long-term difficulties (Morttunen et al 1992). It is described as the end point of a process of escalating distress that fails to be resolved by the person, by his or her closest relations, or by the statutory caring agencies or healthcare practitioners (Aldridge 1998). Maris argues, most convincingly, that the suicidal act is a process, a convergence of many factors over time; it is not an isolated event or the simple product of an acute crisis. He goes on to suggest that a person may have a 'suicidal career' and that understanding this individual career has obvious utility in attempting to interrupt it and bring about an alternative ending. In his preface to his 1981 seminal text *Pathways to Suicide* he states: 'the concept of suicide careers is central' and he continues that nobody 'suicides in a biographical vacuum; life histories are always relevant to the final act of suicide. Suicidal decisions develop over time and against certain social, psychological and genetic or biological backdrops; they are never completely explained by acute, situational factors. '

In a contribution to a later, edited work, Maris (in Leenaars 1991) offered six discrete yet related notions that are captured within the more capacious theoretical view of suicidal careers. We offer a summary of those here:

1. Profiles of completed suicides comprise a range and set of variables (e.g. suicidal ideation, high exposure to suicidogenic populations) and that these sets of variables will differ.
2. Suicidal and life-threatening actions have relevant (and individualized) histories.

3. Reiterating his 1981 statements, Maris points out that suicide deaths are never entirely reactive to present stressors. There is always the presence of suicide career contingencies that mediate reactions to stress (and psychache) and heavily influence the 'here and now moment' of high risk and high lethality.

4. Suicide pathways or careers can vary in duration; thus, suicide lethality can be acute or chronic. (Epidemiological evidence is highly supportive of this notion where data show some people as making multiple serious attempts at suicide over long periods of time, whereas others make one single attempt at a time of high risk/acuity and then make no (recorded) further attempts.)

5. Suicidal pathways predicate the need for models of suicide that encapsulate the whole life-span.

6. These developmental pathway models of suicide should specify both direct and indirect causal paths to suicide.

There are additional implications arising from such a view, and many of these have a high degree of congruence and convergence with other accepted axioms. If one accepts that suicide can be a highly convoluted and complex process that evolves over years (hence the developmental-suicide pathways view), then it must also follow that the 'treatment' of suicide people, or as the authors prefer to phrase, the width and breadth of interventions/programmes that one might use as a carer, is similarly varied, multi-faceted and, most likely, complex. If one accepts the view of pathways or trajectories to suicide, suicide as a process or pathway, then it follows that one has multiple and variable opportunities over time in which one might be able to intervene and make a difference in/to this trajectory.

ALTERNATIVE FORMS AND CONCEPTUALIZATIONS OF SUICIDE THROUGHOUT THE AGES

Suicide as a form of social protest

In her insightful text, Lieberman (2003) points out that suicide can be an aggressive act. Not only an act of aggression acted out upon the suicide victim, but actually an act of aggression towards someone or some other party. Lieberman (2003) refers to the disruptive potential (and therein power) of a person's self-destruction. She writes that death as a weapon can be used to undermine the authority of states, can be used as a form of social protest, and can be used to challenge the very sacrosanct values of societies. Maris et al (2000) perhaps capture such suicides in their description of 'rage-revenge suicides' as they are expressed in suicide notes. While it should be noted that most often this rage (as it is expressed in suicide notes) is couched within problematic interpersonal relationships, for the authors, such descriptions still capture suicide as a social protest. There are examples of such suicides within the literature and within records of suicide cases. For example, two very public examples that are a matter of public record are:

1. In the UK during the mid-1990s, a senior academic from Nottingham University, and a long-time advisor to the former Margaret Thatcher government, took his own life. This tragic event was accompanied by a series

of accusatory and 'damning' suicide letters. Various agencies were unequivocally blamed in these letters for causing (contributing to) this person's suicide. As far as the victim was concerned, he had been ushered into this course of action (and no other) as the only way out; such was the extent of the misconduct and negligence of the agencies he named.

2. A more recent and tragic suicide that might be regarded as a social protest is that of British biological weapons expert David Kelly, and the so called 'smoking gun' as a precursor to the invasion of Iraq. Some contextual detail is necessary, and here we offer a summary of Clancy's (2005) report. In making their case for war against Iraq, British Prime Minister Tony Blair's administration based their argument on the imminent production (and thus potential to use) weapons of mass destruction. Subsequent to this, both the British Broadcasting Corporation and Blair has been put on the defensive as the Hutton Inquiry raised questions about the potentially misleading influence of governments anxious for war. Inextricably bound up with this particular case was top biological weapons expert and government advisor Dr David Kelly, the man who 'blew the whistle' on Prime Minister Blair's government for tampering with crucial dossiers. Kelly, a former nominee for the Nobel Peace Prize, worked in the proliferation and arms control secretariat and was a key advisor to the British government as it prepared dossiers on Iraq's weapons of mass destruction to present to Parliament, which would then decide whether or not to join President Bush and the United States in invading Iraq. Soon after the decision to invade Iraq was sanctioned by the British parliament, not least in part because of the 'evidence' in these dossiers which claimed that Iraq could deploy weapons of mass destruction within 45 minutes, Kelly expressed his concern to journalists that statements made in the dossier were highlighted and exaggerated in order to make the need to go to war seem more urgent. Not surprisingly, on hearing this, Prime Minister Blair set out to squash the statement and whoever had made it. Tragically, Kelly's name was leaked as being the primary source of the journalists' reports and he immediately came under very public and highly critical attack; including the government's assertions that he was *only a civil servant*. Interestingly, the Hutton inquiry shows that British government officials themselves refuted such offensive statements and backed Kelly. Sadly, it is now a matter of record that soon after this public attack Kelly took his own life.

An historical example of suicide as a social protest includes the deaths of the Maze Hunger strike victims who starved themselves to death as a protest against the then British government. Other examples of suicide as a social protest are perhaps typified by 'public immolation': setting oneself on fire in a public place and/or under the gaze of the public. A recent (alleged) example of this was the report of five people setting themselves ablaze on January 23rd, 2001, the day before the Chinese Lunar New Year, in Tiananmen Square, Beijing, China (although it should be noted that some of the Western media were sceptical of the authenticity of this event). A further example of suicide as a form of social protest is that of the Kaiowas tribe in the South American (Brazilian) rainforest. When the colonists arrived in 1940 and started taking their lands, 300 Kaiowas Indians were crammed into a highly constricted area – one surrounded by electrified fencing. Court orders failed to rectify the situation, and between the years 1985 and 1999, 318 members of the tribe killed themselves, mostly by consuming a mixture of insecticide and rum, to try and bring attention to their plight. Lastly, Ulrike Meinhof argued that suicide is the ultimate form of protest; she regarded suicide as a political act, a last resort to preserve one's sovereignty over one's body and life. Interestingly, she later died by suicide while under captivity (as did several of her Red Army Faction comrades). It is interesting to note that suicide as a social protest appears to transcend particular cultures and nationalities.

Suicide to preserve honour and to avoid torture: suicide and the military

There is a well documented association between the military and suicide. First, in considering some of the historical military literature, one can see that suicide sometimes followed defeat in battle. Unless a historian were to search historical documents for evidence of rationales for these vanquished military figures, we can only speculate as to the collection and interaction of particular motives driving these suicides. However, it seems likely that avoiding capture, torture, mutilation, and public shaming and enslavement by the enemy (see for example, Brutus and Cassius, following the defeat of their army at the battle of Philippi; and the mass suicide of rebelling Jews at Masada in 74 AD to avoid enslavement by the Romans). In such instances, suicide appears to be regarded as a better option than the alternative (capture, torture, etc.) and thus has elements of being a positive choice, albeit a 'Hobson's choice'. In such circumstances, suicide would not be viewed as an entirely tragic and nihilistic act. Staying with the example of ancient Roman society, which was, inherent contradictions notwithstanding, the 'height' of what was then regarded as 'civilization', suicide was an accepted means by which honour could be preserved. Those charged with capital crimes, for example, could prevent confiscation of their family's estate by taking their own lives before being convicted in court.

More recently, and perhaps as a result of the historical influence of the Samurai warrior culture, during World War Two Japanese soldiers regarded suicide as an honorable alternative to surrender (and/or capture). This belief was manifest in various forms, including: the continuation of fighting 'to the last man' even in the face of impending defeat rather than surrender; the use of 'Kamikaze' pilots to attack allied ships; the well documented mistreatment of allied POWs. (Indeed, despite the horrific loss of 'civilization' of life following the use of atomic weapons at Hiroshima, the Japanese military still refused to surrender despite the views of Emperor Hirihito notwithstanding.) A more clandestine example of suicide in the military is that of the necessity for 'spies' to carry suicide pills.

CONCLUDING REMARKS

It may be as simplistic and obvious as to be a tautology, but how we, as suicidologists and carers who wish to work with and help suicidal people, frame or conceptualize suicide, will have a huge bearing on how we enact our care, our research, and our practice. In so doing, it might be regarded as paradoxical to begin these conceptualizations without a universally accepted definition of suicide. However, while accepting this possible limitation, it is significant and notable that numerous definitions have been posited and these serve as a useful starting point.

Much academic endeavour has been devoted to the study of the epidemiology of suicide. While it would be prudent to make mention of the methodological and epistemological limitations of these studies, this body of work is valuable and it highlights several key details. It is hard to ignore the compelling data, collected and analysed from around the world, that posits suicide as a major, global health problem; that certain high-risk groups appear to exist (although these are not necessarily consistent over time or place); and that there is an alarming rise in the rate of 'young men' completing suicide in the 'Western world'. Furthermore, these trends over time seemingly stress that despite our sincere efforts at understanding and preventing suicide over the last 50 years, it is fair to say that our efforts have met with (at best) only limited (and perhaps isolated pockets) of success.

Numerous theoretical perspectives exist as a means to explain and understand suicide, although again it would be prudent to recognize that no one single theoretical explanation can account for all the variation documented in suicide. Nevertheless, each particular explanation appears to make cogent points and thus this leads logically to the acceptance of a multi-dimensional model for understanding suicide. Furthermore, Maris' notion of a suicide pathway, trajectory (or career) is difficult to refute and has a very high degree of congruence with multi-dimensional models of suicide. Also, discretion, good sense and forethought requires the acknowledgement of how any explanation of suicide, no matter how comprehensive and accurate it is, may become obsolete as our constructs of suicide change over time; an examination of suicide throughout history indicates that attitudes to and rationales for suicide are rarely static.

Thus, it would be shrewd, and would indicate acumen on the part of the suicidology academe, to purport our contemporary conceptualization(s) of suicide as highly dynamic and contextual. For the authors of this book, however, it seems that our best chance for understanding the obscurity of suicide is to accept the complexity, convolution and intricacy and embrace multi-dimensional, multi-professional models. While this may be re-stating what is already known for some, the relative absence of multi-dimensional, multi-faceted research teams and their associated programmes within the suicidology community perhaps suggests that we have some way to go before actualizing in practice what we recognize and value in theory. Having begun the book with a famous quotation about suicide, it seems synchronous and congruent to also end this chapter with a quotation from another seminal contemporary contributor, Al Alvarez. He states:

> 'The psychoanalytic theories of suicide prove, perhaps, only what was already obvious: that the processes which lead a man to take his own life are at least as complex and difficult as those by which he continues to live. The theories help untangle the intricacy of motive and define the deep ambiguity of the wish to die but say little about what it means to be suicidal, and how it feels.'
>
> A Alvarez in *The Savage God*

Chapter 2

Psychiatric/Mental Health Nursing and Suicide – Policy, Practice and Research

'Improving guidelines and training around procedures like close observation and seclusion can bring appreciable benefits but positive change may not be sustained until underlying attitudes are addressed and consideration given to what P/MH nurses think they should best be doing and are capable of doing . . . Denying the ability (to take one's own life) without addressing the desire must be a major reason why service users find Close Observation unhelpful. Observation without interaction is a cold comfort.'
Peter Campbell 2006, p 272

CHAPTER CONTENTS

INTRODUCTION

Psychiatric/mental health (P/MH) nurses have been intimately involved in the care and management of the suicidal person from the moment that formal healthcare services began to provide services to this population. Further, P/MH nurses are often (but not always) 'front-line' suicide practitioners; they interact with and provide care to suicidal people in numerous settings and at each level of prevention (e.g. primary, secondary, etc.).

Accordingly, this chapter focuses on the extant empirical, theoretical (discursive) and policy literature as it pertains to P/MH nurses and care of suicidal people. It begins by examining the historical and contemporary policy literature from the United Kingdom and Canada. Following this, the chapter draws on literature that outlines (and discusses) the current practice situation *vis a vis* P/MH nursing care of the suicidal person. The chapter then goes on to review the limited empirical literature and in so doing highlights the many gaps in our knowledge base.

PSYCHIATRIC/MENTAL HEALTH NURSES AND SUICIDE IN THE UNITED KINGDOM AND CANADA: THE POLICY CONTEXT

As we highlighted in Chapter 1, given the affiliations of the authors at the time of undertaking the study focused on in this book, we have chosen to focus on data (and information) from Canada and the United Kingdom, where it exists, in an attempt to illustrate how attention to the problem has increased over recent years. This attention has produced a corresponding rise in the associated policy literature, albeit far more so, in the United Kingdom.

In 1990, the document 'Health of the Nation' (Department of Health 1990) was published. Although not specifically a mental health policy document, it nevertheless highlighted suicide as a major cause of death and more specifically showed how certain groups of the population had alarmingly high rates of completed suicide. Perhaps not surprisingly, given the often cited relationship between mental health problems and suicide, people who experience and suffer from mental health problems were highlighted as a particularly high-risk group. Numerous healthcare targets were indicated in this document, one of which was to reduce the number of people with mental health problems who commit suicide by 33%. Whether or not this was a realistic target is a matter of opinion.

It appears that the next health policy document to address the issue of suicide, and it is perhaps noteworthy that this was a mental-health-specific document, was 'Modernising Mental Health Services: Safe, Sound and Supportive' (Department of Health 1998a). Within this document it was stated that suicide was now the second most common cause of death in those aged under 35 years. The broad epidemiological data, methodological limitations notwithstanding, drew attention to a slight overall decrease in the national rate of completed suicide. However, the document also acknowledged that there were still more than 4000 suicide deaths annually in England. Furthermore, the high-risk groups identified in 'Health of the Nation' (Department of Health 1990) had not changed significantly; people experiencing and suffering from mental health problems continued to be identified as one of the highest at-risk sub-groups.

The generic health policy documents continued to draw attention to the problem of suicide; 'Our Healthier Nation: a Contract for Health' (Department of Health 1998b) clearly reiterated the ongoing need to address the problem. Specifically, this document asserted that deaths from suicide (which included deaths resulting from an undetermined injury) should continue to receive attention in an attempt to reduce the rate by a further one-sixth. What this, and many previous policy documents perhaps failed to fully account for (and this largely remains the case) was the highly complex nature of suicide, and concomitantly, the multifarious nature of associated suicide-prevention programmes. This is despite the fact that this complexity had been documented for a number of years (see Maris 1981 for example). Further, the complexity had again been exposed in estimates of population attributable fractions, for both high-risk and population-based strategies. Lewis et al (1997), for example, emphasized that 'broad' strategies designed to reduce the rate of suicide in high-risk populations would, in fact, have only a modest effect on population suicide rates, even if effective interventions are developed.

Soon after the publication of these policy documents, the much touted 'National Service Framework for Mental Health' (Department of Health 1999b) was published. Once more, the problem of suicide in people with mental health problems was highlighted and local health and social care services/communities were exhorted to prevent suicides. However, once more this policy suggested more attention and energy be given to custodial and defensive practices – such as the need for 'safe hospital accommodation', and 'ensuring that clinical staff were competent to assess the risk of suicide'.

While examination of these policy documents shows significant attention (at least at the policy level) to suicide within the United Kingdom, it is fair to say that Canada has lagged someway behind. In 2004, the long awaited Blueprint for a Canadian National Suicide Prevention Strategy was published (Canadian Association for Suicide Prevention 2004); it had been a long time coming. The document acknowledged that, over the last three decades, over 100 000 Canadians had died by suicide, how suicide is indiscriminate – it affects all parts of society – and remains as one of Canada's most pressing public health problems. What is rather startling to realize is how, given the extent and impact of the problem, Canada had not produced a national strategy much earlier. Perhaps this is in part because, in terms of some other more common health problems, suicide remains relatively rare. Yet, when the data are grouped together (e.g. 100 000 people in three decades) and when one considers the 'ripple effect' that each individual suicide has, the scale and severity of the problem become more apparent. The Canadian Association for Suicide Prevention (2004) Blueprint continues to infer that maybe the stigmatized nature of suicide and the ensuing 'silence' in and of itself contributed to the slowness in producing a national strategy. The document purports how many other countries had produced their own national strategies and that now it was Canada's turn.

Interestingly, it is perhaps noteworthy that the Canadian Association for Suicide Prevention (2004) Blueprint does not say anything specifically about P/MH nurses. It may be that P/MH nurses are captured in more broadly described groups (e.g. in goal 4, where the Blueprint refers to developing and promoting effective clinical practice – p 13 – or where it refers to prioritizing intervention services for high-risk groups, p 15). The Canadian Association for Suicide Prevention (2004) Blueprint appears to have particular utility, in the view of the authors, especially when compared to some of the UK (mental health) policy literature as it embraces a more holistic, comprehensive, multi-disciplinary and multi-model approach to addressing suicide (whereas the UK policy literature appears to be more concerned with defensive practices e.g. tightening up observations, more rigorous monitoring of suicidal people). While the Canadian Association for Suicide Prevention (2004) Blueprint does refer to improving risk assessment (and rightly so), it does not stop there; it also emphasizes the need to develop a range of interventions from primary to tertiary prevention, across the full spectrum of the human lifespan and, importantly, encourages the use of multi-method, multi-model studies to help produce a wide range of workable interventions.

Suicide findings reported in the National Confidential Inquiry into Suicide and Homicide by People with Mental Illness (Department of Health 2001)

In concert with the policy literature, the UK Department of Health funded an ongoing epidemiological study to garnish themselves with data. The National Confidential Inquiry into Suicide and Homicide by People with Mental Illness has produced a number of reports, the latest of which (Department of Health 2005) reports a relatively small drop in the suicide rate. While any rise or fall in suicide rate over the short term should be viewed with an appropriate degree of caution, these findings are encouraging. It does, however, continue to reiterate that people with mental health problems remain a disproportionately high-risk group (when compared to the 'general' population).

During the years covered in the inquiry a total of 20 927 cases in England and Wales were notified to the inquiry team. This indicates an annual rate of suicide of 10.0 per 100 000 people. The trend or rate fluctuated during the duration of the study, with a rise being recorded during the first 2 years followed by a fall in most of the 3-month periods since the beginning of 1998. The 'picture' is slightly more alarming in Scotland where the annual rate is 17.3 per 100 000 people.

In England and Wales, 75% of the reported suicides were male, indicating a male-to-female ratio of 3:1. The findings in this study regarding age groups echo earlier reports where the highest number of suicides occurred within the age group 25–34 years, and the next highest in the age group 35–44. The male-to-female ratio was further extended in this highest risk age group where 82% of the suicides were male. A very similar picture was evident in Scotland where 76% were male, giving a male-to-female ratio of 3.2:1. Again, the age group with the highest number of suicides was the 25–34 group, followed by the 35–44. The younger age groups showed a slightly increased difference in the male-to-female ratios where, in the highest risk age groups, 77% of the suicides were male.

Of particular note, the report indicates that 16% of the reported suicide cases in England, Wales, 12% in Scotland and 10.5% in Northern Ireland were psychiatric patients. In these cases, particularly those suicides occurring in the ward environment, the most likely method used was hanging (most commonly from a curtain rail and using a belt as a ligature.) Additionally, around one quarter of these suicide cases died within the first week of admission.

CARE OF THE SUICIDAL PERSON: THE CURRENT PRACTICE POSITIONS

In many parts of the world, P/MH nurses working in in-patient settings currently have 24-hour responsibility for caring for people at risk of suicide (Barker & Cutcliffe 1999, Higgins et al 1998, Hurst et al 1999). Thus, P/MH nurses have, potentially, a major input into the everyday lives of suicidal in-patients. This 'major role' is by no means exclusive to in-patient care. Day Hospitals, Day Care Units and, increasingly, Community Psychiatric Nursing services also perform a major role in the care of suicidal people. Despite this vital responsibility for caring for and safeguarding people at risk of harm, and the potential to offer therapeutic intervention, there is a dearth of evidence and theory to inform nurses in providing such input. Although the phenomenon of suicide is well documented in the literature, very little looks explicitly at the P/MH nursing role, or how the clients perceive and experience the care provided, and its relative merits and demerits. Indeed, despite an extensive search of the relevant empirical and theoretical literature, the authors of this book did not uncover any theory that explains how P/MH nurses care for suicidal people on a day-to-day, hour-by-hour, minute-by-minute basis. Neimeyer and Pfeiffer (1994) offered a similar critique, pointing out the irony that despite the prevalence of suicide, relatively little attention has been paid to training mental health workers in suicide intervention. They added that still less effort has been spent in evaluating the therapeutic effectiveness of such workers.

Some literature does exist, however, and it should be pointed out that most of this is theoretical or discursive, although there is a limited body of empirical work. This, in most cases, is currently the literature that P/MH nurse educationalists are utilizing when preparing course documents and curricula. The most common approach to providing care for suicidal clients can be loosely termed 'observations' (and there are a number of euphemisms for this term – 'specialling', 'close', 'one-to-ones', 'supportive observations' and 'constants' (Barker & Buchanan 2005, Cutcliffe & Barker 2002).

Principal approach: 'observations'

Despite the recognition that suicide is a complex, multi-faceted phenomenon that often requires sophisticated and integrated approaches to care, many texts appear to emphasize the need to 'treat' the underlying affective mood disorder (see, for example, Pritchard 1998). A similar emphasis is espoused by Rawlins (1993, p 281) who suggests that a suicidal client needs to be: 'given anti-depressant medication to elevate his mood and *make him more amenable to treatment* (emphasis added). Electroconvulsive treatment (ECT) is an additional treatment that has proved effective.'

Similarly, authors such as Pritchard (1998) offer some generic suggestions for the care of the suicidal client, e.g. input from a variety of clinicians, improved socio-economic conditions, and social skills training. These broad and perhaps long-term interventions (lithium therapy, antidepressant therapy and ECT) have been shown to be effective in the management of depression. However, and crucially, Gunnell and Frankel (1994) point out that several retrospective reviews of the treatments received by psychiatric patients provided no consistent evidence that these therapies reduce the likelihood of suicide. Furthermore, ignoring the questionable efficacy of these therapies with respect to 'treating' the suicidal client, it is fair to say that they do not appear to say much about the more acute problems facing P/MH nurses when they attempt to engage with suicidal clients.

Some texts, Rawlins (1993) for example, appear to advocate an even more *'masculine and/or defensive'* approach to caring for suicidal clients, when she suggests further 'interventions' include removing harmful items (such as belts, socks) and placing the client on 24 hours a day observations on a one-to-one basis. Rawlins (1993) is by no means the only author to suggest 'close' or 'special' or 'one-to-one' observations as the primary intervention for care of the suicidal client (e.g. Bowers 2001, Libberton 1996, Ritter 1989, Standing Nursing and Midwifery Advisory Committee 1999, Stuart 2001). As a result, for people who are deemed to be 'at risk' of self harm (suicide), harm to others or self neglect, 'observation' has increasingly become the prime focus of care. Furthermore, these levels of observation are most often 'set' by psychiatrists, perhaps with little regard to the demands this might make on nursing staff, emotionally and logistically (Barker & Walker 1999; Mental Health Act Commission and Sainsbury Centre for Mental Health 1997, Moore 1998). In his insightful study of special observations of suicidal psychiatric in-patients, Duffy (1995) reported similar findings where he noted that, in each case studied, special observation was formally prescribed by a doctor, indeed, usually a junior doctor. Perhaps more importantly, he also reported that, despite the special observations being prescribed by doctors, they were always carried out by P/MH nurses, and as a result special observation had come to be specifically a nursing activity. Consequently, Duffy (1995) reported the nurses' discomfort with being identified (by some disciplines) as custodians rather than therapeutic practitioners. While individual units, wards, health units, hospitals and Trusts may well have their own policy on 'close or special observation', these policies share key commonalities. Further, an international comparison of these observations policies shows remarkable congruence and similarity. One such example of a 'close observation' policy is provided in Box 2.1.

Observation: safe and effective?

Despite the continued emphasis on 'observation' as the *modus operandum* for the care of the suicidal person, it is increasingly being called into question and as a result alternative models of care are being considered. Although nurses' use of observation and 'specialling' has been in evidence for almost 25 years, the therapeutic value of such approaches to care has long been questioned. The practice of observation was developed as a means to inform medical staff of the status of the patient (Barker & Cutcliffe 1999, Nolan 1993). It served the function of assuring the 'absent' doctor of the physical

Box 2.1 Example 'Close Observation' policy

1. The level of observation should be determined by risk assessment, be a constituent part of the plan of care and be recorded in medical/multi-disciplinary notes.
2. Observation levels are prescribed by the responsible medical officer.
3. A nurse may increase the level of observation following a risk assessment (but must inform the RMO and the multi-disciplinary team as soon as possible).
4. The planned delivery of the close observations will be organized by the nurse in charge of the shift; and recorded on an observation rota. This rota will identify the member of staff delegated to undertake observations for a specific time span.
5. All staff must be clear of their specific responsibilities and sign to confirm that they have completed the span of observation.
6. Close observations should not be carried out by the same nurse for a duration of longer than 2 hours.
7. When passing on the responsibility for close observations to another nurse, the following must be discussed; the level of observation, the nature of the risk, restrictions of patient's movement, any special consideration, any relevant information concerning the patient's mood or behaviour, and ensure that the level of observation is understood.
8. Every effort should be made to promote a therapeutic relationship with the patient; minimizing the distress caused by the process.
9. The patient should be informed of the level of observations.
10. Significant others, where confidentiality allows, should be informed of the level of observations.
11. The allocation of staff to close observations should take into account aspects of the individual's needs, e.g. gender, ethnicity.

Adapted from the Standing Nursing and Midwifery Advisory Committee (1999).

safety of the patient. Yet as statistics for suicide in in-patient settings (Department of Health 1999b, 2001) and the first author's own research experience of attending over 90 suicide or open verdict inquests illustrate (see Cutcliffe & Ramcharan 2002), observation as a caring practice is a woefully weak intervention. For between 20 and 33% of the suicides committed while in-patients, many of these were 'under' levels of observation (Department of Health 1999b, 2001). Where observation policies exist, there is a great deal of inconsistency in the interpretation of these (Department of Health 1999b, 2001) and yet further problems with actioning or carrying out these observations. Now it needs to be acknowledged that the Standing Nursing and Midwifery Advisory Committee (1999) report, and the work arising out of this report, may go someway to addressing some of these problems (although this remains to be seen). Nevertheless, it also needs to be acknowledged that additional problems remain.

Key evidence resides in the service users' experiences of close observation and the limited body of evidence in this substantive area is predominantly consistent. Evidence from Newcastle (Barker & Walker 1999) and York

(Fletcher 1999) indicates that while being 'under observation' clients (or mental health service users) felt neither safe nor supported. One user summed up the experience succinctly when he stated: 'some do closes (observation) nicely. They talk to the patient like a friend and still carry on with their other duties. But others are like robots; when the patient moves they follow like zombies.' (Barker & Walker 1999, p 56). Whereas, a service user in Fletcher's (1999) study indicated: 'They didn't actually ask me if I was feeling suicidal. Just went everywhere with me.', and a member of staff stated: 'I would be happy to say to somebody "don't try anything because I am going to be with you all the time and I don't want that responsibility on me." '

More recent evidence from Oxford (Jones et al 2000) and Bradford (Dodds & Bowles 2001) lends further support to this position. Jones et al (2000) found that most of the research subjects in their study did not like the experience of being observed, found it intrusive, and that some nurses did not talk to the users at all during the observation period. This was found to be a particularly negative experience. Similarly, in Dodds and Bowles' (2001) attempt to dismantle observation and move towards a more 'care'-orientated system, the following findings were established. Incidents of deliberate self-harm reduced by two thirds, violence and aggression reduced by over a third, staff sickness fell by two thirds, absconding declined by half, and there was no increase of suicides during the corresponding period (18 months). Importantly, they state: 'the effect on patient care has been striking: patients are more engaged with their named nurses, better informed and more involved with their care.' (Dodds & Bowles 2001).

Stevenson and Cutcliffe (2006) used a Foucaultian analysis to illustrate that 'observations' is contingent upon many factors, the least of which is the suicidal person's need(s). As a result it perhaps comes as no surprise that the therapeutic value of such approaches to care is being questioned.

The 'Who' question

Inextricably linked to the alleged value (or otherwise) of observations is the matter of who carries them out. Extensive shortages of P/MH nurses across the United Kingdom has led to a reliance on 'bank' or 'agency' staff. In the study of Gournay et al (1998), the authors found that bank nurses provided between 23.6 and 36.3% of the staff compliment and the authors quite rightly went on to condemn this practice as unacceptable. While such figures vary in different sites across the UK, this pattern is by no means exclusive to London or to the United Kingdom (Dodds & Bowles 2001). Compounding this situation, in many (most) parts of the country, observation is carried out in the main by support staff, bank/agency staff and students (Barker & Cutcliffe 1999). That is not to suggest that trained P/MH nurses never carry out observations, but the majority of the observations are not carried out by trained P/MH nurses. The issue of observations being carried out by 'practitioners' other than trained/experienced P/MH nurses is by no means limited to the United Kingdom. In the study undertaken by Cardell and Pitula (1999, p 1067), these authors state that: 'the individuals who provided constant observation were 13 hospital staff members, including registered nurses and mental health technicians, and seven minimally trained lay workers or sitters.'

Unfortunately, Cardell and Pitula's paper does not provide a clear indication of exactly how many registered P/MH nurses provided observations, but it is clear that some of the observations were conducted by technicians and minimally trained workers or sitters. Similar and somewhat disturbing patterns are to be found in Canada. In witnessing care of the suicidal person in several Canadian hospitals, the first author found that that such 'care' is still largely driven by custodial rather than therapeutic concerns. In some hospitals, security guards rather than P/MH nurses carry out the 'observations' of the suicidal person. In others, suicidal people are simply placed in seclusion rooms and the observations are carried out *apropos* a modern day version of Bentham's Panoptican; that is, there is no human–human connection what-so-ever and the suicidal person is 'monitored' by means of a closed-circuit TV system (Holmes at al 2004). Having witnessed such practices, the first author declared: 'even though such a situation leaves me feeling very uncomfortable, in some ways, this 'care' delivery model may be more honest than those care delivery models which claim to provide more than custodial care, yet in reality, often don't.' (Cutcliffe 2003, p 256).

Consequently, there is evidence to suggest that observation is widely and invariably regarded as a low-skill activity, often carried out by support staff (rather than registered P/MH nurses), or by bank or agency nurses who, by their transient nature, have only limited knowledge of the person. Such a position, according to Dodds and Bowles (2001) is counter-productive, contributes little in the way of assessment and treatment within acute wards (Moore 1998), or to the development of new approaches to acute inpatient care (Mental Health Act Commission and Sainsbury Centre for Mental Health 1997). Indeed, this situation leaves P/MH nurses in reactionary, custodial roles (Higgins et al 1998) and despite the rhetoric of 'supportive observation', the P/MH nurse is often construed as a custodian, if not a doorman.

A need to change the focus?

Crucially, the complexity of people at risk of suicide or self-harm is axiomatic. Such people need highly specific, and sophisticated, forms of care. There is a growing recognition that the P/MH nursing care of people who are at risk of suicide or self-harm needs to re-focus on a more manifest form of care and support, rather than upon tightening up the policing strategy of observation. However, there has long been a consensus, at least in the USA, that given its covert nature, suicidal intent imposes – by virtue of its invisibility – a negative emotional impact on P/MH nurses. Given the demands of caring for suicidal people, Hamel-Bissel (1985) argued that P/MH nurses need many years of experience before they could manage successfully the professional stress involved. Clearly, the emotional impact or 'labour' of caring for suicidal people, the sophisticated and complex forms of care and the unique challenges that such clients present, necessitates the need for regular clinical supervision. This would provide the opportunity for the nurses to receive appropriate, regular and restorative support necessary to enable them to continue working with such people. Such structured reflection not only assists the unique challenges to be met but, additionally, offers the nurse an opportunity to learn and develop the knowledge, skills and attitudes needed to care for such individuals.

Certain critical incidents (e.g. dealing with violence and aggression, engaging with suicidal clients) may even indicate the need for formal debriefing sessions and further additional forms of support. However, such clinical supervision and formal support mechanisms have not always been in place. Indeed, the absence of support systems is likely to give rise to P/MH nurses whose high stress levels preclude them from further therapeutic engagement with suicidal clients. Thus, the authors would argue that engaging with suicidal clients reiterates and reinforces the need for P/MH nurses involved in such care practices to receive appropriate clinical supervision (we return to this crucial point in Chapter 9).

Summary of the 'observations' approach

Thus, in summary, observation as a means of intervention for people who are suicidal:

- is a system that was designed originally to inform (absent) psychiatrists and now, at least in part, is concerned with meeting the needs of the healthcare organization; it is essentially and primarily a 'defensive' practice;
- fails between 20 and 33% of those people it is supposed to protect (and these numbers are even more alarming when one considers the number of people who go on to harm themselves once the 'observation' restrictions have been lifted;
- is a crude, 'custodial' orientated form of intervention to meet the highly complex, convoluted and sophisticated a care needs of this client group;
- is operationalized in the main, despite the recognized complexity, by transient (bank/agency) staff or support workers with minimal training;
- does little (if anything) to address the route of the client's problems which led him/her to feel suicidal in the first place; does little or nothing to address the suicidal person's psychache; and
- is highly stressful for the P/MH nurses who participate.

Studies that investigated current service provision: primarily 'observations' related literature

It is perhaps ironic to note that even though the use of 'observations' (in various forms and guises) appears to be the *modus operandi* for care of the suicidal person at the moment – and currently this can be seen to represent the dominant discourse – there is very little empirical evidence that exists to support the use of observations for suicidal people; and the literature that does should be regarded with an appropriate degree of caution given the methodological limitations. One of the first things to be noted is that no study has even tried to examine whether being under certain levels of observation actually reduces the number of suicide attempts; there is no randomized control trial that has attempted to compare units with close observation against units without constant observation. As a result, the only 'comparative' data that we have in this area conceivably comes from evaluatory 'studies' following on from changes in service delivery (see Bowles et al 2002, Dodds & Bowles 2001).

As stated above, in the only published paper of such practice development that the authors could locate (Dodds & Bowles 2001), following the dismantling of observation and moving towards a more 'care' orientated system, the following findings were established. Incidents of deliberate self-harm reduced by two thirds, violence and aggression reduced by over a third, staff sickness fell by two thirds, absconding had declined by half, and there had been no increase of suicides during the corresponding period (18 months). Furthermore, although not an empirical piece, in the discussion paper arising out of this 'study' a number of compelling testimonies are evident, as well as further confirmation that removing observations led to *a reduction – not an increase in – suicide rates*. Interestingly, one of the most compelling testimonies for removing observations comes not from a P/MH nurses, but from a psychiatrist. In referring to the introduction of formal observations for suicidal people, Dr Phil Thomas purports: '(P/MH) Nurses were no longer expected to talk with patients, but to observe them . . . but the introduction of nursing observations signified a cultural change, a shift from a philosophy that valued human contact, to one in which facts and enumeration were of greater importance. A phenomenon that gains pace, as our attraction to tick-box assessment testifies. . . . If formal observations were introduced for defensive reasons, then in my opinion they also created a voyeuristic mentality, an intrusive disentangled gaze on human suffering. Something was lost when nursing observation became the norm on inpatient units' (Bowles et al 2002, p 256).

As with many other reports of the client's experience's of 'being under' observation, powerful, highly provocative and gripping statements that have an unavoidable spontaneous validity for anyone who has seen such practices are provided by service users in Bowles et al (2002). Indeed, not that we wish to prejudice any ensuing debate, but after hearing such account we wonder why any P/MH nurse would advocate *for* observations. Diane Hackney states she was told being under observations would: 'give me someone to talk to about my problems. It would keep me safe. It would help me get better. In fact, the absolute opposite happened . . . Most of the staff I got lumbered with did not, could not or would not make even small talk with me, let alone discuss my illness . . . it always amazed me that the least experienced staff were given the most distressed patients to work with . . . I often felt guilty about wanting to move from one room to another as this was regularly met with a lot of tutting and heavy sighs from my nurses. It appears that all this activity was just too much for them now that they had got settled in one spot or were deeply entrenched in a magazine or book. . . . There have got to be ways of helping a person feel safe and supported without reducing them to victims of voyeurism and seriously eroding away their basic human rights.' (Bowles et al 2002, p 256/257).

A small number of studies have attempted to investigate both the clients' and the P/MH nurses' experiences of observations, and have similarly tried to extrapolate that the experience is either therapeutic or not therapeutic. While we welcome such research activity, we regard the findings with a degree of caution (as a result of the methodological limitations) and further, regard such papers as providing parts of the overall picture (and evidence); not all of it. For example, tragically, the experiences of those people who were under observations and still managed to complete their suicide will never be available to us. Even the most junior researcher would thus recognize that this will skew any sample of clients who have been under observation. Cardell and Pitula (1999) attempted to investigate suicidal inpatients' perceptions of observations. In what they claim was a grounded theory study, although it appears as though there is evidence of methodological slippage; especially slipping into a small-scale survey, participants reported both therapeutic and non-therapeutic aspects of observations. The therapeutic aspects were described as observer intentions, optimism, acknowledgement, distraction, emotional support, and protection. Non-therapeutic aspects were described as lack of empathy, lack of acknowledgement, lack of information, lack of privacy, invasion of personal space, and confinement. When one examines this paper in more detail, it becomes clear that it is certain attitudes and practices of the P/MH nurse within the (or during the) observations that appears to be experienced as therapeutic, and not the being observed per se. For example, Cardell and Pitula (1999, p 1068) note that 'therapeutic observers' were described as caring, helpful, and hopeful; having observers acknowledge or recognize them as unique and meaningful human beings was fundamental to the development of a helpful therapeutic relationship with the observer. Indeed, one participant reported: 'I think having somebody speak to you makes a more positive experience. I mean a million times more positive. It's beyond qualification how important it is. Just come in and talk to you.' Similarly, another client statement emphasized the affirmation of his self-worth and stated: 'You know, it is simple compassion. When you feel that someone is there, it means a lot. . . . It's like someone cares.'

Unfortunately, Cardell and Pitula (1999) report that these experiences were by no means universally encountered, for 30% of the sample, being under observations did little to alleviate hopelessness, and actually increased their anxiety or aggravated their dysphoria. A staggering 55% perceived a lack of acknowledgment from observers; these perceptions sometimes overlapped with perceptions of a lack of empathy. In keeping with other empirical work and with many other anecdotal reports, these behaviours included observers reading books, appearing distracted or disinterested in the participant, and acting like the participant was a burden. Lack of privacy was again documented, to the extent that 25% of the clients reported disruption in their daily hygiene and elimination. Most worryingly, in the view of the authors, 10% of the participants informed researchers that they lied about their degree of suicidality in order to hasten the termination of constant observation. The implications of this finding are staggering. This intervention, allegedly used to help people not complete suicide actually leads to purposefully misleading information, false assessments of suicidal risk and adds another layer of psychache to the already psychologically burdened suicidal person.

Fletcher's (1999) study provides some illuminating findings, the methodological limitations notwithstanding. The author claims to have used an ethnographic approach but there appears to be evidence of methodological slippage and the method described has much in keeping with the tenets of a phenomenological approach. Further, while inherently concerned with culture, Fletcher's findings didn't say very much directly about the 'culture of observations', his findings appeared to say more about the experiences of observing and being observed. However, it was particularly refreshing to see such 'honest' data regarding the use and purpose of 'constant observations' (and thus perhaps speaking indirectly to the concept of a culture of observations). An example of such honesty is the author's finding which acknowledges that, despite the rhetoric of 'supportive observation' (Barker & Cutcliffe 1999), the use of 'constant observations' clearly has an element of serving the needs of the organization rather than the needs of the individual. A further strength of the paper, according to the members, was the author's attempt to obtain data from, and subsequently induce a theory from the clients' perspectives. This is a body of evidence that remains mostly absent. Therefore, a study such as this, despite its limitations, might be regarded as a useful contribution to this under researched substantive area.

The pilot study undertaken by Jones and colleagues (Jones et al 2000) found similar equivocal findings; the experiences of the sample were mixed. Interestingly, and in keeping with the above mentioned studies, the participants who found the experience of being observed positive, *were those who said their nurses engaged* (our emphasis) with them, leading to a greater sense of security and support. A further study, reported in Cutcliffe and Ramcharan (2002) was carried out in the late 1990s. The study aimed to investigate potential reasons why people committed suicide; as a result the research team interviewed the family and friends of over 70 suicide victims. Initial contact was made with the families at the Coroner's inquest, and the subsequent interviews were carried out at a negotiated time, usually within 6 months of the victim's death. During the inquests additional data were recorded, and the case files were examined. Even given the limitations of the method and the inconsistent nature of the case files, it was evident that between 20 and 33% of the completed suicides occurred while the client was 'under' some level of formal observations (e.g. more than the standard level).

A more recent study (MacKay et al 2005) makes a number of interesting claims, one of which being skilled or more experienced P/MH nurses were more likely to undertake observations than junior, untrained, sitters or bank nurses. This is a peculiar claim to make given that the authors claim they obtained a purposeful sample of six experienced P/MH nurses, each of whom had specific experiences of undertaking observations. It may also be regarded as somewhat incongruent to have a quantitative finding (e.g. who is more likely to carry out observations) from a study that intended to have: 'A specific focus on staff perceptions . . . and will explore and describe elements of this (observations) process' (MacKay et al 2005, p 465).

Furthermore, while there may be merit in the study undertaken by MacKay et al (2005), caution should be exercised when considering the results as they actually refer to what nurses *say they are doing* and to the nurses' *beliefs about the effects of their* interventions; what the nurses may actually be doing could be different. Also, there are no data from clients as those who experience the observations; thus it is mostly speculative as to the effect.

Studies that have attempted to articulate the suicidal person's experience and the nurses' experiences of care for such people

A small literature exists that attempts to describe the experience of feeling suicidal and the subsequent experience of care. Samuelsson et al (2000) used a qualitative method to interview people who had attempted suicide. The participants stressed the value of being well cared for and being understood. Similarly, Carrigan's (1994) study examined the psychosocial needs of patients who have attempted suicide by overdose. Davidhizar and Vance's (1993) study of the management of the suicidal patient in a critical care unit stressed the need for the nurses to consider their own attitudes towards suicide, in order that they can ensure that they do not distance themselves from the client. They emphasized the importance of communicating acceptance, given that suicidal clients are highly vulnerable to responses from care givers, and stated the value in hearing the clients when they are ready to talk.

The study of Talseth et al (1997) produced similar findings. These authors reported the value of compassion and emotional identification when caring for the suicidal client, in addition to the trust that is built through regular contact between client and the P/MH nurse. Further, they described how P/MH nurses attempted to demonstrate care for suicidal clients and thus confirmed rather than criticized the client's emotions and feelings. Lastly, Talseth et al (1997) described how the P/MH nurses who cared for suicidal clients ensured they listened to the clients. The later work by Talseth et al (1999) purported the value of P/MH nurses initiating contact with suicidal clients, and attending to clients' basic needs (including the value of physical contact with suicidal clients). Also, according to Talseth et al (1999) P/MH nurses must accept suicidal clients' feelings, be open to these people and have time for them, and listen without prejudice. Similarly, Long and Reid (1996) and Long et al (1998) asserted the value and necessity for the P/MH nurse to offer unconditional positive regard and empathy to suicidal clients, and pointed out the therapeutic value of hearing and empathizing with the suicidal client.

Some extremely interesting insights are provided by those papers that offer first hand accounts of suicidal experiences and feelings (e.g. Aldridge 1998, Crook 2003). Walen (2002) refers to excerpts from her diaries to illustrate some of the key experiences while feeling suicidal. Some of these first hand accounts make reference to depression spanning many years through her formative and adult years. She describes, in detail, her detachment from those close to her and the need to be able to communicate her feelings. She urges professionals to allow people time to talk about their experiences as being able to express feelings is pivotal in lifting the isolation experienced by a person in suicidal crisis. Crook (2003) confidentially interviewed 30 teenagers about their experiences of suicide and revealed themes they thought to be important in their lives. These were based around five themes, which bear strong similarities with Walen's diary accounts. These included needing to belong, having friends to share their perspective, the value of family, the need for a purpose in life and finally power over their emotions.

More recently, Sun et al (2005) describe a simplistic process of care for suicidal Taiwanese psychiatric in-patients. They outline a four-stage model: holistic assessment, provide protection, provide basic care and provide advanced care. While they do not appear to explain how, for example, restraining or secluding suicidal people helps address suicidal ideation or suicidality per se, their emerging theory emphasizes a more custodial driven approach to caring for suicidal people than that described in the above cited literature (or more custodial than the findings reported in the present study). Interestingly,

Sun et al (2005, p 281) conclude: 'The emergent findings ... indicated that psychiatric nurses should have the skills and qualities required to provide advanced care for suicidal patients, the compassionate art of nursing was generated as the overarching principle ...'.

SUMMARY

Paradoxically, while it can be seen that suicide continues to represent a clear public health issue for both Canada and the UK, neither nation can be complacent where care of the suicidal person is concerned. While there is a substantial literature that focuses on suicide, there is a distinct paucity of literature that informs the P/MH nurse about the more acute problems facing nurses when they attempt to engage with and provide care for suicidal in-patients. There is clear absence of literature that informs the P/MH nurse of how to provide care day-by-day, hour-by-hour and minute-by-minute, for the suicidal person.

It is evident that 'models' of care for the suicidal person in both Canada and the UK still emphasize the notion of making the person 'physically' safe. Such models appear to be based on the premise of maintaining the person's safety while they are in 'suicidal crisis' and then gradually reducing the level of observations; perhaps simultaneously administering anti-depressant medication. Patterns of admission and discharge of suicidal clients clearly imply such a premise, where in (most often), suicidal clients have very short lengths of stay.

Also, and importantly, when one examines the literature that supports the use of close observations or makes claims that being 'under' close observations is therapeutic a more enlightening finding is clear. It is not the experience of being under observations per se that produces any therapeutic benefits – it is the P/MH nurse's attitude of care/concern that makes a difference. It does need to be acknowledged that there is an increasing amount of dissent regarding the hegemonic position of observations and as a result, the body of literature pertaining to P/MH nursing care of the suicidal person is far from harmonious, containing as it does a number of papers that critique and subsequently challenge the value of observations as the *modus operandi* for care of the suicidal person (Barker & Buchanan 2005, Barker & Cutcliffe 1999, 2000a, Barker et al 1999, Cutcliffe 2003, Cutcliffe & Barker 2002, Dodds & Bowles 2001, Fletcher 1999, Gibbs 1990, Higgins et al 1998, Moore 1998).

Some sections of this chapter have been reproduced with kind permission from:

Mental Health Practice (RCN Publishing)
Journal of Psychiatric and Mental Health Nursing (Blackwell Publishing)

Chapter **3**

Research Methods and Suicidology

'It means that our best route to understanding suicide is not through the study of the structure of the brain, or the study of social statistics, or the study of mental diseases, but directly through the study of human emotions described in plain English, in the words of the suicidal person.'
Edwin Shneidman 1997, p 24

'Conceptualisation is the core of Grounded Theory . . . conceptual theory is concerned with the generation of concepts that have enduring grab.'
Barney Glaser 2001, p 22

CHAPTER CONTENTS

INTRODUCTION

Contemporary health care is synonymous with the often touted phrase 'evidence-based'. This apparently simple phrase has multiple meanings and several implications for people who use the concept. While we acknowledge these multiple meanings, here we consider the phrase to imply that practitioners, wherever possible, need to have an established evidence base to support their clinical practice. We also recognize, especially as we adopt and embrace a pluralistic approach to knowledge generation, that evidence comes in many forms, including the pivotal form of 'empirical evidence'; evidence derived from research. Additionally, a crucial element of the evidence-based practice 'movement' is that said evidence, irrespective of the type or form, should not automatically be taken at 'face value'; the evidence should be subject to critique and critical reading. Accordingly, it is necessary for researchers to include details of their method and design. In addition to providing some of the contextual material that will enable thorough critique, it is also customary practice for researchers to describe their research design and methods. There is a case for arguing that this may be even more important for qualitative studies. Since methodological precision is a hallmark of high-quality research and determining the credibility of research findings relies, in part, in critiquing the rigor of the method, it is prudent, if not required, that we include text that describes both, 'what we know' as a result of this study, in addition to 'how we know'. Hence, this chapter describes and explains our research design and method; it provides the methodological context necessary for understanding the findings.

HISTORICAL AND CURRENT METHODOLOGICAL TRENDS IN SUICIDOLOGY

Given the worldwide increase in suicide rates and the multi-dimensional costs of suicide (e.g. emotional costs, societal costs, economic costs), it is not surprising that a substantial literature exists. Much, although not all, of this can be described as empirical literature; reports of research studies that attempt to add to our understanding of suicide and suicidology. An examination of the contemporary efforts to understand suicide contained within this literature indicates that the current emphasis is clearly on quantitative methods, clarifying characteristic symptoms, symptom clusters, risk factors, establishing causal links and identifying clinical phenomena associated with the presence of suicidal behaviour (Silverman 1997). Indeed, according to one of the most pre-eminent contemporary suicidology scholars, Dr Ronald Maris, there is a distinct bias in favour of funding biomedical suicide research. This funding trend has also been noted by the CIHR/Health Canada (White 2003) Working Party on Suicide Research wherein it was observed that suicide research (in Canada) is firmly rooted in the traditional scientific paradigm where a concern with prediction and control is placed in the foreground. This focused study of factors associated with suicide has been well documented during the last 60 years. Not surprisingly, this has resulted in a body of knowledge that is far from unified and unequivocal, containing, as it does, many unresolved controversies (Silverman 1997). Encouragingly, two issues that appears to have a very high degree of consensus within the scientific academy of suicidologists are:

1. Suicide is a multi-dimensional, complex phenomenon, it needs to be recognized as such and interventions/strategies (and associated research activity)

should reflect this (Maris 1997a, Silverman 1997, Task Force on Suicide in Canada 1994, White 2003). Indeed, Maris (1997a) offers a cogent argument for embracing the 'biopsychosocial perspective' for studying suicide.

2. There is growing recognition and support within the scientific academy of suicidologists, for the idea of a 'pathway(s)' or 'trajectory(s)' of suicide (Maris 1981, 1990, Shneidman 1997). In this conceptualization, the developmental-existential perspective of suicide is purported. Suicide is posited as an end point to a person's 'psychache', the psychological pain resulting from multiple distresses occurring in one's life (Shneidman 1997). It is predicated as a person's inability or refusal to accept the terms of the human condition (Maris 1981), as the end point of long-term difficulties (Morttunen et al 1992). It is described as the end point of a process of escalating distress that fails to be resolved by the person, by his or her closest relations, or by the statutory caring agencies or healthcare practitioners (Aldridge 1998).

Despite this extant theory, Maris (1997a, p 57) argues that: 'we still have little solid knowledge about the social dynamics or "suicidal careers" of eventual suicides'. He qualifies his argument with the example that while we know a high percentage of completed suicides tend to be socially isolated at the time of death, how they came to be that way is less understood. Drawing on a United Kingdom and Canadian specific example in order to illustrate this argument, we know that a high number of completed 'young' male suicides in the United Kingdom had a statistically significant relationship with alcohol misuse; what ushered them into this misuse and resultant suicidal ideation is less well understood. (This correlation between completed suicides and alcohol use/misuse is a common finding in many studies examining risk factors in First Nation Canadians as well.) Further, we also know that 'young' Canadian males choose more 'lethal' methods of suicide than their female counterparts; how they came to choose this method and what experiences ushered them to this choice are less well understood.

QUALITATIVE RESEARCH WITHIN SUICIDOLOGY: A 'NEW' APPROACH?

As stated previously, recent studies or programmes of research in the area of suicidology that have used a qualitative method or methods, are relatively absent from the literature and their utility has been questioned by some. In the light of this emphasis, even though the authors are positive advocates for qualitative methods (where methodologically indicated), it may appear as foolhardy to construct an argument for augmenting the current research emphasis within suicidology by suggesting that we embrace more qualitative methods. That being said, a more thorough examination of the historical extant research literature pertaining to suicidology indicates the significant contribution that has been made by studies and programmes using qualitative methods.

Durkheim's 1897 study of suicide (re-published in 1951) has long being recognized for its seminal contribution and, for some, is regarded as the beginning of formal study of suicide. Interestingly, Durkheim's work included the use of qualitative approaches. Subsequent to this, and more recently, another noted suicidology scholar, Jack Douglas, helped to create the research method of ethnomethodology in sociology during his tenure at the renowned Los Angeles Suicide Prevention Centre. His important 1967 contribution, *The Social Meanings of Suicide*, questioned some of the methodological trends that were dominant at that time. Just like Durkheim, Douglas (1967) questioned founding the scientific study of suicide on vital or official statistics. In place of focusing on external and constraining facts, such as suicide rates, Douglas (1967) argued that we need to observe the subjective accounts or situated meanings of actual suicidal individuals. Further, he made the impassioned case that the way to discover the meaning of suicide is to observe the statements and behaviours of individuals actively engaged in suicidal behaviours.

Following on the heels of this work, Professor of Psychiatry Ron Maris' undoubted contribution to suicidology, emanating from the Centre for the Study of Suicide in South Carolina, has culminated in the production of what he terms a biopsychosocial perspective of suicide (Maris 1992, 1997a, b). This model not only necessitates the need for methodological pluralism within suicidology, but simultaneously advocates the need for interdisciplinary study of suicide. He states: 'Because suicide is not one kind of behaviour, the explanation of suicide cannot be by a single factor or the province solely of any one professional discipline or specialty area.' (Maris 1997a, b, p 53).

Notably, this need for multi-professional, collaborative research in suicidology was reiterated in the Health Canada/CIHR (White 2003, p 55) descriptive summary of suicide-related research in Canada. This paper pointed out key gaps in the extant suicide research literature and stated: 'Educational research and investigations about suicide from a nursing or social work perspective are also rare, despite the relevance of suicide to these professions'.

Furthermore, perhaps the outstanding suicidologist of his generation, Edwin Shneidman, is convinced that suicide is a state of mind and not necessarily a quantifiable, biological phenomenon (Shneidman 1997). According to Silverman (1997), Shneidman makes persuasive arguments that suicide is a consequence of the failure of the individual (and society) to address pain and frustrated psychological needs (the 'psychache') of the suicidal individual. Shneidman continues: 'it means that our best route to understanding suicide is not through the study of the structure of the brain, or the study of social statistics, or the study of mental diseases, but directly through the study of human emotions described in plain English, in the words of the suicidal person' (Shneidman 1997, p 24).

More recently, in Montreal, February 2003, the Canadian Institutes for Health Research and Health Canada, organized and sponsored a Workshop on Suicide-Related Research in Canada. Specific objectives of this workshop were:

- to review the range of suicide-related research in Canada and internationally;
- to identify and establish themes that will guide suicide-related research over the next 10 years; and
- to support multidisciplinary collaboration in research and knowledge translation.

As a result of the review, the workshop highlighted a number of key points regarding the situation of the current suicide related research endeavours in Canada. They acknowledged that while much work has been done, there remain many unanswered questions, and that the emphasis has been, and remains, on quantitative studies. Accordingly, the workshop concluded that more emphasis should be given to qualitative studies and this was reflected in the methods attached to each of the six identified research themes. The six themes identified were: (in no order of priority):

1. Data systems: improvement and expansion.
2. Evidence-based practices.
3. Mental health promotion.
4. Multi-dimensional models for understanding suicide-related behaviour.
5. Spectrum of suicidal behaviours, including suicide attempters.
6. Suicide in social and cultural contexts (White 2003).

Further, with respect to themes 3, 4 and 6, the clear methodological emphasis arising from the workshop was a move towards qualitative methods, particularly the use of phenomenological, hermeneutic, and narrative studies. Lastly, it should be noted that the requirement for methodological pluralism and within that, an acceptance of the utility of qualitative methods within suicidology, has been highlighted repeatedly recently (Cutcliffe 2005a, Goldney 2002, Lester 2002).

Thus, in summary of this section, it can be seen that there is a well established historical 'track record' within suicidology of studies using a variety of qualitative methods. Far from being inappropriate to this area of study, many leading suicidologists have made the case that what is currently lacking are contemporary qualitative studies; these individuals purport that by focusing exclusively on quantitative methods, many of the key questions and answers will remain beyond our collective grasp. Accordingly, the next section of the book describes the particular qualitative method (and research design) that we used for our study.

SELECTING THE APPROPRIATE RESEARCH METHOD: DESIGNING OUR STUDY

Choosing or selecting the most appropriate method for any study is a critical issue and one that necessitates serious and deliberate consideration. The axiomatic position for such selections is that the choice of method is driven by two key questions, namely: (a) what is the precise research question and (b) what do we (as an academe) already know about the phenomenon? It is well documented that a qualitative method is usually used when little is known about a phenomenon (Morse & Field 1995). Further, the hypothetico-deductive approach to knowledge generation indicates that one firstly induces a theory (especially where no extant theory exists) before then proceeding to test the theory, deductively. In addition, qualitative methods are particularly useful when describing a phenomenon from the emic perspective (i.e. from the native's or participant's point of view).

The authors had noted that here was a dearth (if not an absence) of existing empirical literature, and the authors wanted to examine how (if at all) P/MH nurses cared for suicidal people; how they helped (if at all) move the suicidal person from a death-orientated to a life-orientated position. Furthermore, the authors were concerned with obtaining data from the perspective of the person who experienced the suicide 'crisis'; as Shneidman (1997) advocates, we wanted to access the human emotions described in plain English, the words of the suicidal person. As a result of these methodological considerations the authors decided that a qualitative method was clearly indicated as most appropriate for this study.

The next issue facing the authors was selection of the most appropriate qualitative method. According to Morse and Field (1995), the differences between the major qualitative methods are: (a) the specific questions they answer, (b) the different methodological requirements and (c) the different types of results they each produce. Consequently, the authors needed to consider the following questions:

1. What method would be most appropriate to the question: how do P/MH nurses care for the suicidal client?
2. What are the methodological requirements? – e.g. participants, data collection methods?
3. What type of results are required?

In response to question 1

The practice of providing care for the suicidal client clearly involves at least two people and also occurs over a period of time. Accordingly, it can be seen that the authors were concerned with studying a process; a process between clients and formal carers Thus, we needed to select a research method that is concerned with uncovering and understanding basic (psycho)social processes between clients and formal carers. Thus, a grounded theory method was indicated as the most appropriate (Glaser 1978).

In response to question 2

The authors needed to obtain data from the groups of people involved in this psychosocial process. Furthermore, the authors could obtain the richest data by means of interviews (e.g. 'can you tell me about the psychosocial process?') or observation (looking for evidence of the psychosocial process). Thus, a grounded theory method was indicated (Glaser & Strauss 1967).

In response to question 3

The authors needed results that would describe and explain the psychosocial processes of care for the suicidal person. We wanted to induce a specific theory for P/MH nurses that would guide them in providing care, day-by-day, hour-by-hour, minute-by-minute for this client group. Thus, a grounded theory method was indicated (Morse & Field 1995). Accordingly, the authors decided that a grounded theory method would be the most appropriate method for this study. According to Glaser (1992), it would have been inappropriate to carry out an extensive review of the literature prior to commencing data collection. However, having being involved in the care of suicidal people for many years, the authors were already familiar with some of the literature in this substantive area, such as it is. (The literature that the research team was aware of, however, indicated that there was a distinct paucity of empirical work that described and explained how care of the suicidal person is undertaken. As a result, the research team is empirically confident that the induced theory is an accurate representation of the psycho-social process between the participants and is not an imposition of their own agenda.) Thus, it was inappropriate (or impossible) to attempt to unlearn or try and forget this literature. It is therefore methodologically accurate to describe the method used in this study as a modified grounded theory.

An overview of modified grounded theory

As stated earlier, the clear methodological trend in suicidology currently is quantitative methods; deductive, and verification studies. It should be noted that grounded theory is concerned with generating theory (Glaser & Strauss 1967). Its basic and central theme is generating theory from data that is systematically obtained from social research consequently grounded theory is an inductive process. It is a both a method and a methodology for developing or inducing a theory; a theory that should provide clear enough categories and hypotheses that explain and aid understanding of the basic social (or psychosocial) process being studied. The theory evolves from the data during the process of the research, and does so continuously. In that, unlike many other methods, the researcher does not commence with existing literature but begins with an identified area of study. Then, as data are collected, the process of constant comparative analysis occurs whereby each item or label of data is compared with every other item or label. Glaser and Strauss (1967) stress that this strategy of comparative analysis within the induction of grounded theory puts a high emphasis on: 'Theory as process, that is, theory as an ever-developing entity, not as a perfected product'. It concentrates on the interactional processes at work within the world, provided by the perspective of the participants, and these perspectives are then replaced by theoretical conceptualisation (Glaser 1998, 2001, Smith & Biley 1997). Grounded theory usually occurs when there is little or no research into the research subject or area. Consequently, research questions in grounded theory (if present at all) are markedly different to research questions postulated at the start of a deductive study. The question needs to be flexible and open-ended enough to allow freedom for the theory to develop (Glaser 1998, 2001).

The crucial difference between grounded theory and deductive approaches is its emphasis on theory generation and development (Glaser 1998, 2001, Glaser & Strauss 1967). It is a way of thinking about and conceptualizing data, in order to induce theory that is grounded in the reality of the research process. That is the theory generated is developed through interplay with the data collected during research projects. The theory can be seen to originate from the 'ground level', from the social world where the data originates. Grounded theory researchers construct theory from the data rather than applying a theory constructed by someone else from another data source, the theory thus remains connected to or grounded to the data, and in that way grounded in reality, the specific reality of where the data originated from. As a result, a grounded theory should therefore 'fit' the situation being researched. To sum up:

> 'A well constructed grounded theory will meet its four most central criteria: fit, work, relevance, and modifiability. If a grounded theory is carefully

induced from the substantive area its categories and their properties will fit the realities under study in the eyes of subjects, practitioners and researchers in the area. If a grounded theory works it will explain the major variations in behaviour in the area with respect to the processing of the main concerns of the subjects. If it fits and works the grounded theory has achieved relevance. The theory itself should not be written in stone or as a "pet", it should be readily modifiable when new data present variations in emergent properties and categories.'

Glaser 1992, p 15

KEY FEATURES/ELEMENTS OF GROUNDED THEORY

There are four principle features of grounded theory, firstly, is its emphasis on theory generation, not theory verification. It produces two basic kinds of theory, substantive or formal theory. Grounded substantive theory is theory that has been developed for a substantive or empirical area of social enquiry, for example client care (This is the type of grounded theory that will be described in this book, i.e. a modified grounded theory for the substantive area of care of the suicidal person). Grounded formal theory is theory that has been developed for a formal or conceptual area of sociological enquiry, for example deviant behaviour. Glaser and Strauss (1967) asserted that substantive theories are usually induced from the data and formulated first and then these substantive theories are followed by formal theories, through additional comparison with data obtained from areas other than the substantive (for a more detailed description see Glaser 1978, 1998). A grounded theory should have several elements that are generated by comparative analysis; these are conceptual categories and their properties, hypotheses or generalized relations among the categories. Each of these elements are defined:

- Categories – a conceptual element of the theory that stands by itself (Glaser & Strauss 1967, p 36).
- Property – a conceptual aspect or element of a category (Glaser & Strauss 1967, p 36).
- Hypotheses – a suggested, not tested, relation among categories and their properties (Glaser & Strauss 1967, p 39).

The second principle feature is theoretical sampling, which involves jointly collecting, coding and analysing the data and deciding what data to collect next and where to find them, in order to develop the theory as it emerges. Glaser and Strauss posit that this method of sampling is a radical shift away from the methods used when attempting to generate theory, whereby the limits, scope and origins of the sample are pre-determined. A grounded theorist, however, still needs a starting point, and Glaser and Strauss described this starting point as the researcher beginning the research with a partial framework of local concepts, which designate a few principal or gross features of the structure and processes under study. Unlike studies that are designed to verify theory, theoretical sampling within grounded theory does not cease once a pre-determined number of sample units have been accessed, theoretical sampling ceases once the categories are saturated. The researcher has achieved category saturation when no additional data are being found whereby the researcher can develop properties of the category.

The third key feature is the constant comparative method. This involves comparing incidents. The researcher codes his data and then compares each of these coded incidents with one another and then codes these incidents into as many categories of analysis as is possible in order to let the categories emerge from the data. Then the researcher integrates categories and their properties. As coding continues, the constant comparative units change from comparing incident with incident, to comparing incidents with the emerging categories. These take the form of clarifying the logic, taking out non-relevant properties, and integrating details of properties into the major outline of interrelated categories. Further the theory undergoes the process of reduction. This enables the researcher to formulate the theory with a smaller set of higher level concepts and hence delimit the theory in its terminology and text.

The fourth key feature is termed theoretical sensitivity, which contains two processes which are pivotal to that end, namely, searching for and discovering the core variable and the need for all grounded theories to have a temporal dimension or identified stages. In explaining the importance of the core variable, Glaser (1978) posited that searching for patterns in the generation of theory revolves around a core variable; without an identified core variable, a grounded theory is incomplete and limited in its application. The second process crucial to theoretical sensitivity is that of grounded theories having a temporal dimension or stages. The core variable will have two or more clear emergent stages and these stages should differentiate and account for variations in the pattern of behaviour. Since, in Glaser's (1978) view, a process is something which occurs over time and involves change over time, the variations over time within the core variable can be explained by the stages.

SELECTION OF THE SAMPLE AND DATA COLLECTION

A total of 20 participants were selected using the principles of theoretical sampling; wherein the choice of whom/what to sample was driven by the emerging findings rather than any apriori constructed sample selection criteria. Thus, each subsequent choice about whom to sample is a deliberate choice designed to help expand, delimit and densify the emerging theory. All participants belonged to the substantive group of 'people who have received formal mental health care for a suicidal crisis after making a serious attempt on their life.' Such clinical delineations were assessments made by the expert clinical judgement of the client's consultant psychiatrist. (Note, as stated in Chapter 1, precise definition of a genuine suicide attempt is an imperfect and problematic matter. Nevertheless, some attempt had to be made to differentiate between genuine suicide attempts and non-genuine suicide attempts. Accordingly, we deferred this assessment to the expert clinical judgement of the responsible consultant psychiatrist. As a result, if after 'admission' and assessment the consultant psychiatrist deemed the person's attempt to be a genuine attempt to end their life, then we regarded this as someone eligible to be potentially included in our sample.) None of the participants were cared for by the authors or any of the research team. The formal mental health care was provided in various settings (e.g. in-patient, day patient or community based clients), and at several graphical locations in the United Kingdom. During the analysis of the data, no theoretically relevant differences according to the person's gender; age, race, theological and/or cultural backgrounds or beliefs emerged, therefore, no such variations in the sample were pursued. The length of the formal care received varied between participants, though the extent of variation was not large, the care episodes lasting between 1 and 7 days as an inpatient, and several months as a community based client. The frequency of visits from Community P/MH nurses following discharge was variable. All participants, however, received 'treatment' from P/MH nurses; all had initial input/treatment from a psychiatrist, some had input from additional formal mental healthcare professionals (e.g. Social Workers) but the day-to-day, hour-by-hour, minute-by-minute care was provided only by P/MH nurses.

In keeping with Glaser and Strauss' (1967) directions for sample selection, the authors began with individuals from the same substantive group. These individuals were former clients who had received care for a 'suicide crisis' as 'community clients'. Following this, the emerging theory indicated that there might be merit in increasing the differences in the sample. Namely, the emerging theory had started to indicate that the particular physical and social environment might have an influence on the person and that adjusting the environment to make it as stress free as possible could be a therapeutic intervention. As a result, we accessed former clients who had received care for their suicidal crisis as in-patients. Following this, the emerging theory indicated that the research team needed to sample formerly suicidal clients who had received care in a 'Day Hospital' or 'Day Unit' setting, because there may have been particular therapeutic value for suicidal people in some of the activities that occurred on Day Units. Also, in accordance with Glaser and Strauss' (1967) directions, the research team sampled individuals from several geographical locations within the South Yorkshire and the Newcastle areas.

Data were collected by means of a semi-structured interview, interviews taking place in a quiet room, either within the informant's home, or within the counselling centres. Each interview was audio-taped, and transcribed verbatim. The interviews lasted between one and two hours and the authors began with a very loose structure; as the tentative theory began to emerge the interviews became more focused. Thus, when entering interview one, the only written question the authors took into the interview was: 'If you could begin by telling me about your recent experiences, perhaps you could say something about what brought you into contact with the services and what, if anything, the P/MH nurses did during your care episode'.

This capacious statement became more focused during subsequent interviews. When entering later interviews, the written questions/key issues, indicated by analysis of the previous transcripts, that the authors took with them included:

'How did the Community Psychiatric Nurses (C.P.N.s) make you feel secure, what did they do?'
'How did you get a sense that they were bothered about you?'
'Could you talk us through a typical day at the day hospital then?'
'And what about the P/MH nurses, what did the P/MH nurses do if anything?'

'Some of the previous people we have interviewed have talked about perhaps having a nurse physically close to you, and maybe even following you
around. Perhaps if they had decided that you were something of a threat to
yourself. Did you encounter any of that?'

'Did that give you some hope?'

'So being asked to challenge it at that time wasn't right for you?'

'So what was it that nurse 'X' was doing at that time for you?'

'So what was the difference with nurse 'X's' technique? What was different about nurse 'X' that you did get somewhere? Was it immediate?'

Furthermore, in keeping with Glaser's (2001) methodology, in earlier interviews the authors used predominantly 'exploration' questions. As the data
were subsequently analysed, and the theory began to emerge, we used a combination of 'exploration' and 'confirmation' questions. As the theoretical categories began to become more saturated in the later interviews, we used
predominantly 'confirmation' questions.

DATA ANALYSIS

It is important to note, that given the process of the constant comparison
method within modified grounded theory, the stages of data collection and
data analysis do not occur in a linear sequence, they are cyclic in nature.
However, for the purposes of describing how we operationalized our
method, the process of analysis is described in stages. The first stage involves
transcribing each interview. Following this, Glaser and Strauss' (1967) process
of open coding is applied. This entailed examining the text line by line and
identifying the processes in the data. Each of these identified processes is then
coded (on individual index cards) and these were termed 'labels' or 'incidents' or 'codes'. This process of coding is termed 'substantive coding'
because the labels codify the substance of the data, often using the very words
of the participants themselves. Next, we attempted to discover the key psychosocial processes in the social scene, from the point of view of the participants,
hence each label was then compared with every other label and these were
assigned to clusters or categories according to obvious fit. This allowed a tentative conceptual framework to be generated from the preliminary categorization of the data. Further, the authors devised a tentative heading for each of
the preliminary categories. This was accomplished by examining common
themes, concepts evident in each of the categories, or alternatively by identifying if there was an underpinning process or theme. For example, in the context of this research, several statements mentioned 'finally getting the chance
to talk', 'being listened to by the nurse' and 'feeling that someone was understanding the participant's point of view'. Hence this preliminary category
was termed 'Talking about one's experiences and feeling understood'.

The next stage of the analysis saw the development of the tentative framework. This was achieved by using two major steps to both expand and densify
the emerging theory, these were: reduction and selective sampling of the data.
The authors examined the preliminary categories and perceived links; discovered 'umbrella terms' under which several categories fit, as a result of comparing each preliminary category with other preliminary categories to see
how they clustered or connected. The umbrella term can thus be seen to

encompass several preliminary categories. For example, several of the preliminary categories appeared to contain, or allude to, a similar process – namely, a process that suggests that the nurses would engage in subtle, implicit challenging of the person's suicidal constructs. Hence the developed category 'Implicitly challenging suicidal constructs as a result of encountering contrary experiences' was induced. Simultaneously, further comparison with more data then helped the refinement of these concepts and variables. Additional selective data were collected for the specific purpose of developing the hypotheses and identifying the properties of the main categories (epitomizing the practice of theoretical sampling). The final stage was dominated by two phases, theoretical coding and comparison with the extant literature; though it should be noted that given the paucity of extant literature, there was not a great deal to compare with. Concepts were compared with more highly developed concepts, and these were compared with more data. This enabled the production of the sub core variables and core variable; it enabled the authors to conceptualize and represent the theory in its most simple form; in other words, it enabled the production of a parsimonious theory.

The procedure described was complicated, but also enhanced, by having a team of researchers, each of whom was involved in the data collection and analysis (John Cutcliffe [JC], Chris Stevenson [CS], Sue Jackson [SJ] and Paul Smith [PS]); although Professor Barker was intimately involved in the early stages of the study, he did not undertake any data collection or analysis. It is important to set out the team's approach as a means of establishing the fidelity to the particular form of modified grounded theory chosen. The first interviews were substantively coded by JC. As this occurred, the list of codes was shared with the rest of the research team and this helped to orient further interviews – in relation to what was asked of whom. Thus, theoretical sampling was established. (See above for examples of the evolution and development of the interview questions.) As the interviewing progressed, the expanding codes were circulated among team members and there was further discussion regarding the coding itself and categorization of codes. Given the geographic distance between team members, the discussions took place via telephone and video conferencing, email and occasional face-to-face meetings. The discussion was fuelled by theoretical memos made by team members and, again, this directed the process of future interviews. Nearing the point of data saturation, the team devoted time to looking at every label, composition of each category (in the interest of constant comparison); description of each category and to teasing out the processual dimensions of categories. This built upon JC's initial conceptualization of the temporal dimensions of the theory. Every theoretical and analytic choice was considered. Where there was disagreement between the team, debate ensued until the analytical choice with the most 'grab and fit' was arrived at. It cannot be over stated that the aim was not to reach a consensus that reflected an absolute 'truth', in the spirit of verificationism. That is to say, the categories were not being validated through the agreement of team members, neither were the team members seeking nomothetic generalizable 'truths' arising out of the findings. Rather, the discussion tapped the creative imagination of the team members. It threw up different interpretive/conceptual possibilities, which allowed the development of denser theory that could account for similarities and differences.

Hence, conceptual development was achieved in part, as a result of these debates. The results had immediate 'grab and fit' for the team members.

As the team refined categories, memo'ed and conceptualized, it became apparent that data saturation had occurred. However, three further interviews were conducted as a means of checking that no new processes were identified by the participants. Selective sampling also drove the interviews. Specifically, the participants were asked directly about aspects of the developing theory, increasing the density of description. Having established the psychosocial processes in the suicide scene, each of the research team took categories belonging to each stage and engaged in category reduction. Relevant literature was woven in, although there was not much pre-existing work to weave into the theoretical matrix. This meant that parallel literature needed to be explored to see whether or not it could hold up a conceptual mirror to the emerging modified grounded theory. This is described in more detail in later chapters. The stages were circulated amongst the team to read and comment. The process facilitated the elaboration of the core variable.

ETHICAL CONSIDERATIONS

Ethical issues in this study were addressed in keeping with an approach that has been described as being more fitting for studies with an emergent design, namely the 'ethics as process' approach (Cutcliffe & Ramcharan 2002, Ramcharan & Cutcliffe 2001). Accordingly, while ethical approval was obtained from both Local Research Ethics Committees where the study was undertaken, ethical issues were repeatedly revisited throughout the duration of the study. Thus, consent was re-visited and re-established with interviewees, a 'safety net' of services for interviewees was provided in the unlikely event that they needed additional formal healthcare support following the interview and relationship endings with participants were protracted rather than sudden. Interestingly, no interviewee reported or showed any evidence of being harmed by the interview process.

Chapter 4

Re-connecting the Person with Humanity: the Core Process

'While there is nothing inherently wrong with descriptive level studies we, as a scientific community, need to do much more with our current research than describe. Indeed, the most illuminating qualitative findings go far further than description, they interpret, they explain; they solve problems.'
Cutcliffe & McKenna 2004

'It helped me not commit suicide, even though I was thinking about it, because I knew there were people (the P/MH nurses in Community Assessment Team) who were bothered about me and didn't want me to.'
Interview N7

CHAPTER CONTENTS

INTRODUCTION

In this chapter we provide a 'broad, brush stroke' description and an explanation of the core (psycho)social processes that the P/MH nurse uses in order to provide meaningful care for the suicidal person, and in so doing, describe and explain the 'core variable' (Glaser & Strauss 1967) of this emerging theory. The central or core variable of this theory is 'Re-connecting the person with humanity'. This core variable is able to account for all the codes and categories and so provides an explanatory whole to all coding. It explains, in a parsimonious form, how the participants in this study solved their key psychosocial problem. In other words, in asking the question 'How do psychiatric/mental health nurses move the suicidal person from a death orientated position to a life orientated position?' our findings indicate that P/MH nurses achieve this through re-connecting the person with humanity, and through all the processes contained within this conceptualization. Re-connecting the person with humanity describes a three-stage process of healing; each having its own conceptual heading, and these are shown in Box 4.1 and diagramatically represented in Figure 4.1.

Furthermore, as stated in the previous chapter, the cyclic and parallel processes of data collection and analysis within the grounded theory method meant that extant literature, such as it was, could be woven into the emerging theory when theoretically indicated. Accordingly, the authors begin this chapter by outlining the required conceptual level that a core variable should have. Following this the authors describe and explain the existential state that the formerly suicidal participants in this study found themselves in during their suicidal experiences. This existential state is illustrated by drawing on the extent, related literature and through the process of conceptualization. The chapter then describes the core variable. After reading this chapter, the reader should be able to understand both the empirical background and theoretical development of the core processes involved in meaningful caring work with suicidal people. As a result the findings should have more credibility, more spontaneous validity (Kvale 1996) and more, to paraphrase Glaser (1978), fit and grab.

Box 4.1 Sub-core variables category composition

'Reflecting an image of humanity' (stage one)
Experiencing intense, warm, care-based human to human contact.
Implicitly challenging suicidal constructs as a result of encountering contrary experiences.

'Guiding the individual back to humanity' (stage two)
Nurturing insight and understanding.
Supporting and strengthening pre-suicidal beliefs.
Encountering a novel interpersonal, helping relationship.

'Learning to live' (stage three)
Accommodating an existential crisis, past, present and future.
Going on in the context set by the existential relationship with suicide.

Figure 4.1 Re-connecting the person with humanity.

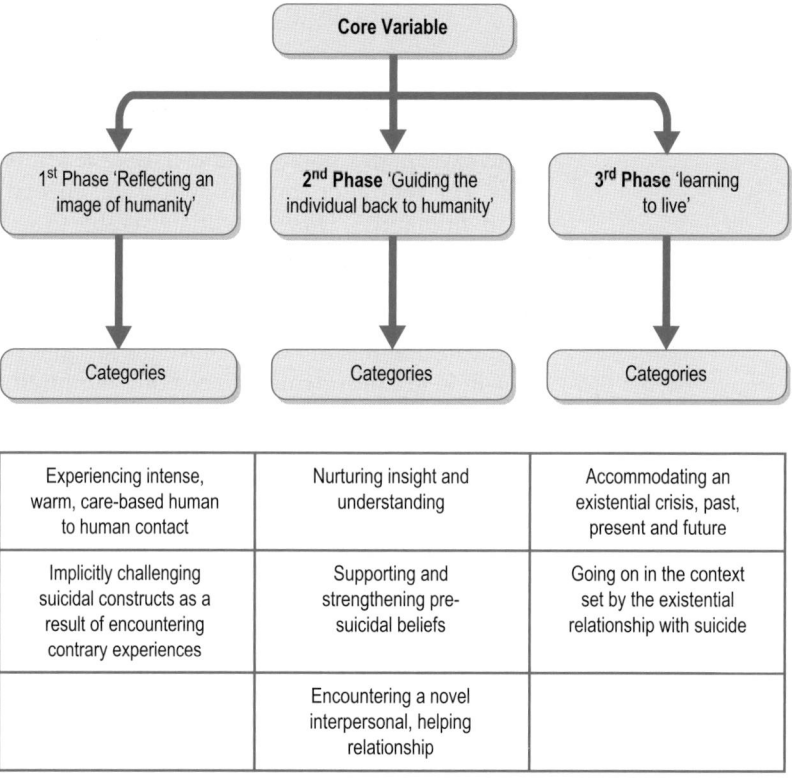

Categories	Categories	Categories
Experiencing intense, warm, care-based human to human contact	Nurturing insight and understanding	Accommodating an existential crisis, past, present and future
Implicitly challenging suicidal constructs as a result of encountering contrary experiences	Supporting and strengthening pre-suicidal beliefs	Going on in the context set by the existential relationship with suicide
	Encountering a novel interpersonal, helping relationship	

THE REQUIRED CONCEPTUAL LEVEL OF A GROUNDED THEORY

In keeping with the tenets of grounded theory, a grounded theory must include conceptualization; Glaser (2001) has stated recently that conceptualization is the core of GT. Conceptualization (*vis a vis* conceptual theory) referring to the generation of concepts that are abstract of time, place and people; generating concepts that have 'enduring grab' (Glaser 2001, p 22).

Conceptualization involves the naming of psychosocial patterns that are grounded in the research and need to be at the 'third level' of conceptual analysis (Glaser 2001, p 22). According to Glaser (2001, p 30) 'In detailing the contrasts to follow I will try to show how the confusion between description and conceptualization results in a weakening of GT by and for description and a defaulting of GT to standard Qualitative Data Analysis'.

Furthermore, this third level of conceptual analysis is perhaps more synonymous with core variables, where the parsimonious theory should contain no more than the fewest conceptual elements. Such third level conceptualizations require the qualitative researcher to 'move beyond the words' of the participants.

'Expert qualitative researchers go beyond the words, see past the obvious, access the underlying and the hidden, and enlanguage the often present yet invisible process/culture/experiences.'

Cutcliffe & McKenna 2004, p 130

Accordingly, rather than being replete with individual quotes from the participants, the core variable of a grounded theory should provide a conceptual overview of the theory; it should not drift into descriptive capture. It should, however, be able to account for all the codes and categories and provide an explanatory whole to all coding. It should explain, in a parsimonious form, how the participants in this study solved their key psychosocial problem.

THE SUICIDAL PERSON: EVIDENCE OF 'DISCONNECTION' IN THE EXTANT LITERATURE

Suicide and social integration

Since the beginning of the formal study of suicide, the relationship between the individual person's sense of connection (and its associated synonyms) and the resultant increase in suicidality has been posited and discovered with conspicuous regularity. Furthermore, it is interesting to note, especially in the light of Maris' (1997a, b) comments regarding the requirement for adopting a biopsychosocial perspective for studying suicide, that this sense or experience of 'disconnection' is manifest in a variety of ways; it is a multi-dimensional, multi-faceted existential experience. (It is worthy of note that Maris's views are echoed throughout the international academe of suicidologists wherein a multi-dimensional and multi-disciplinary approach to the study of suicide is now, for many, regarded as *de rigueur*.)

For some, the formal study of suicide began with Emile Durkheim's classic work *Le Suicide* (1897/1951). Durkheim's central claim was, perhaps counter-intuitively, that the apparent highly personal and individual act of suicide was in fact driven or even determined by social, external (and constraining) facts. Moreover, he was clear in predicating the causal relationship between the individual person's sense of social isolation (what he termed *egoism*) and the eventual suicide. For Durkheim, the suicide rate had an inverse (though variable) relationship with the person's sense of social integration. He posited three 'types' of suicide: egoistic, altruistic and anomic. Highlighting the then differences in rates of suicide of people who claimed to be Protestant, Catholic or Jewish – differences which continue to be reported in some studies – with rates recorded as highest in the Protestant population and lowest in the Jewish population, Durkheim asserted that these differences in rate occurred as a result of the different degrees of 'unity, solidarity and integration' that existed within these groups. He argued that, for example, in response to the external hostility directed towards people who held the Jewish faith, this helped establish and maintain strong community ties of thought and action and also discouraged divergence. To use contemporary suicidology parlance, these community ties thus acted as a very powerful 'protective factor'.

A further interesting proposition from Durkheim was that there was a relationship between the degree of free thought or free inquiry and the rate of suicide. To paraphrase, when a group 'permits' or encourages free thought, the result will be increased knowledge and Durkheim argued, a corresponding increase in suicide rates (since free inquiry can result in as much sorrow and despair as it can happiness). It is worthy of note that in Durkheim's view, the protective influence of religion and religious beliefs do not arise as a result of the particular theological view of suicide (e.g. suicide as a sin against God), but occurred rather because religion is a society; it enhanced the person's sense of integration, belonging and connectedness. Thus, Durkheim's famous reference to a 'coefficient of preservation'; and his conclusion that the stronger the integration of the religious community, the greater its preservative value.

Interestingly, Durkheim's views of the preservative value of societies were not comprehensively supported by the rates of suicide in other societies, although some supporting evidence was reported. For example, Durkheim produced evidence to show that marriage acted as a preservative factor *for men but not for women*, also when the marriage partner died, then the loss of the preservative influence of this 'society' was marked.

While we wish to include a caveat here that Durkheim did not define what he meant by his use of the term 'social integration', the authors of this book argue that there is an apparent, noticeable and palpable relationship between social integration and a sense of connectedness. Synonyms for the word 'integration' include: inclusion, incorporation, combination, assimilation, merging and merger – whereas antonyms include: separate, exclude and reject. Similarly, the synonyms for connection include: bond, relationship, link, association, union, tie, network and bring together. Thus, it is clear that integration and (re)connection appear, at the very least, to share an etymological connection; we will return to and develop this connection throughout this chapter. Though, for the authors of this book, the relationship between this connectedness and integration transcends the uni-dimensional view of 'social' connectedness/integration; again, this is further explored below.

Interestingly, while one has to recognize and acknowledge the 'vintage' of Durkheim's work, contemporary findings lend much support to the notion of social integration and the resulting sense of connection as a distinctive protective factor against suicide. Perhaps the better modern examples of this include suicide rates within Northern Ireland, and the context of political instability and associated acts of terrorism – known or referred to colloquially as 'the troubles' (McGowan et al 2005, p 400). McGowan et al (2005) accessed official suicide statistics in Northern Ireland for the period 1966–1999 and found that nearly 7000 people had died prematurely over these years. A highly significant inverse correlation ($P < 0.01$) was found between the annual number of suicides and deaths caused by terrorist activity. This correlation was found to exist across both genders. McGowan et al (2005) conclude that the strengthening social bonds that occur as a result of experiencing 'the troubles' – or to paraphrase, the increased sense of being connected to one's social community arising from the sense of being persecuted or being under attack – act as a significant protective factor against the risk of suicide.

Social isolation, loneliness and suicide

A further experience(s) that is perhaps synonymous with a sense of disconnection is that of social isolation and loneliness. A sizeable literature exists that indicates a positive correlation between a person's sense of isolation and/or loneliness and increased risk of suicide; furthermore, this isolation is manifest in a variety of forms. While noting its vintage, a seminal paper on the role of social isolation and suicide was written by Trout (1980). Trout's conclusion, which if subsequent studies (see below) are anything to go by, still has meaning and significance in the 21st century. Trout's systematic review of the literature concluded that social isolation seems to be related to suicidal behaviours in a direct and fundamental way.

More recent work, and work with specific populations who can and do experience a high degree of social isolation, reiterates and supports Trout's findings. One such population is the elderly, and more especially, the widowed. A well established literature purports the risk of suicide is increased in the widowed (see, for example, Fawcett et al 1987, Goldstein et al 1991, Motto et al 1985, Powell et al 2000, Wenz 1977). Indeed, again accepting the vintage of the study, Wenz concluded that in addition to the social psychological factor of anomie, it was the *actual social isolation* and the *future social isolation* (our emphasis) that were the key factors in widows who lived in urban sub-areas.

Loneliness, which clearly has an association with social isolation, has often been identified as having a correlation with suicide and increased suicide risk; furthermore these associations are not limited to one group of the population. In the 'Western World' the elderly population continue to have an alarmingly high of rate of suicide, and similarly, report high levels of social isolation and loneliness (due to a wide range of variables). (We are mindful of both (a) the sometimes pejorative nature of the term 'elderly' – however, this is the term used commonly in the literature – and (b) that it would be simplistic to refer to one homogeneous group called the elderly.) Not surprisingly, the association between loneliness in the elderly and suicidal ideation/behaviour has been reported (Osgood 1991, Osgood & Brant 1990, Tatai & Tatai 1991). While it would be rash or hasty to suggest a direct causal link between social isolation, resultant loneliness and all suicides in this population, it is evident that a link exists. A larger number of studies and, as a result, a more developed body of knowledge refers to loneliness in young people, most often high (senior) school and College (University) students. At first glance, such findings might seem counter-intuitive given that the physical proximity to other people in such places is often close. Yet the findings are consistent, over time and place, in showing a significant link between loneliness and suicide in these populations (Bonner & Rich 1987, Garnefski et al 1992, Rich & Bonner 1987, Rich et al 1992). More recent evidence indicates that during a cluster of suicides at New York University in 2003, students reported the sense of isolation and stated that there wasn't a social atmosphere. Interestingly, this mix of academic pressure and social isolation has been reported in other schools and universities and is clearly a high-risk mix.

Loneliness has been discovered to feature as one the principal factors that contributes to suicide in several other studies, for a variety of nationalities (Lavigne-Pley 1987, Stravynski & Boyer 2001, Torre et al 1988). In the most recent of these studies, Stravynski and Boyer (2001) found strong associations, in a population-wide survey, among suicide ideation and different ways of being lonely and alone. They further noted that the prevalence of suicide ideation increased correspondingly with the degree of loneliness. These associations were found to almost the same degree in males and females.

Further evidence points to the association between social isolation and increased suicide risk. Suicide rates are frequently found to be higher in rural and remote regions than they are in densely populated regions. Drawing on the example of British Columbia, Canada, when compared to their urban counterparts who live in the south of the Province, health outcomes, including rates of suicide, are markedly worse (British Columbia Vital Statistics Agency 2001, 2002). The epidemiological picture is further complicated across Northern British Columbia wherein some geographical areas have very low (almost non-existent) suicide rates and others have suicide rates well above the national or provincial average. Annually collected data indicate that there were 192 completed suicides in 2001 within the geographical area covered by the Northern Health Authority. Moreover, of this number 136 (71%) occurred within the North West Health Authority region area, a region with the significant majority of the population living in remote and rural areas. Similar findings have been reported in other countries – see for example, recent epidemiological data from Australia, Wales, and the USA. While acknowledging the social isolation that can occur with remote and rural populations, the authors urge a degree of caution here; it may well be that there are other variables that 'contribute to' the high rate of suicide in these regions. Nevertheless, it is worthy of note.

A further population group who are perhaps synonymous with experiencing isolation are the homeless. While accepting that homeless people may (or may not) belong to a social group of their 'peers', it similarly needs to be accepted that the homeless person is likely to be isolated from his/her family, friends, and various support systems. Eynan et al (2002) undertook a study to examine the association between homelessness and suicidal ideation and behaviours; their findings were disturbing. Out of their sample of 330 homeless people, 61% reported suicidal ideation and 34% had made an actual attempt. Of particular support of the relationship between isolation (as experienced through homelessness) and suicidal ideation, their study also found that childhood experiences of homelessness were found to be associated with suicidal ideation.

Accordingly, one can conclude with a degree of empirical confidence that social isolation/loneliness, in a variety of forms and individualized experiences, clearly has been identified as having a correlation with suicide and increased suicide risk. Furthermore this link has been observed across several specific population groups as well as different nationalities.

Suicide, psychache and (dis)connectedness

Edwin Shneidman is often regarded to be the pre-eminent suicidologist of his generation and is credited with fashioning the contemporary formal study of suicide and thus creating the scientific field 'suicidology'. Shneidman's central premise appears to be that suicide is inextricably linked what the term he coined, *'psychache'* (original emphasis):

'Stripped down to its bones, my argument goes like this: In almost every case, suicide is caused by pain, a certain kind of pain – *psychological pain* (original emphasis) or "psychache". Further this psychache stems from thwarted or distorted psychological *needs*. (original emphasis).

Shneidman 1997, p 23

While Shneidman qualifies his remarks and acknowledges that there are certainly exceptions and further that the topic is a very complicated business and thus *ipso facto* is unlikely to be explained by a straightforward single causative relationship, he makes a compelling case for considering the relationship between the presence and influence of pervasive and pernicious individualized psychache. He continues:

> 'even though I know that each suicidal death is multi-faceted event; that biological, biochemical, cultural, sociological, interpersonal, intra-psychic, logical, philosophical, conscious, and unconscious elements are always present – I retain the belief that, in the proper distillation of the event, it's essential nature is *psychological* (original emphasis). That is, each suicidal drama occurs in the *mind* of a unique individual. (original emphasis)'
>
> Shneidman 1997, p 23

Accepting the cogency of this premise, it is then worth considering how psychache might affect a person's sense of disconnection. Furthermore, if we invert this, if we accept the possibility of an existential state of disconnection, it is worth considering how this might affect a person's psychache.

It is now accepted as axiomatic that the experience of pain has emotional as well as a physical component. This multidimensionality of pain is encountered not only in the nature of the pain experience itself, but also in *the effects* of experiencing pain. Furthermore, while a range of pain-relieving interventions can alleviate the physical sensation of pain (Carr & Mann 2000, Schofield 2005), there is a large and well established body of extant literature that indicates how pain can wear the person down; make him/her feel emotionally exhausted, anxious, depressed, and/or overwhelmed. Indeed, there is a growing body of work that refers to the 'depressant' effects that chronic pain can have on people (Mossey & Gallagher 2004, Tesch et al 2004, Turk et al 1995). Additional psychological and social effects of pain have been reported and these are summarized in Box 4.2.

Also, there are narrative based accounts that people with pain may well be afraid to tell anyone about their pain. The concern most often reported is that such individuals worry that they will be labelled a 'complainer'; it is the person's lot to endure or suffer in silence. This is despite the copious and

---

Box 4.2 The psychological and social effects of pain

- Being less able to function
- Feel tired and lethargic
- Loss of appetite and/or nausea
- Not being able to sleep, or having one's sleep interrupted by pain
- Experiencing less enjoyment and more anxiety
- Becoming depressed, anxious, or unable to concentrate on anything except pain
- Feeling a loss of control
- Having less interaction with friends
- Being less able to enjoy sex or affection
- Feeling that one is more of a burden on family or other caregivers

convincing evidence that refers to the subjectivity of pain. Indeed, the often cited maxim in nursing is that pain is what the person says it is and when the person says it is! The extant 'pain' related literature has also illustrated that the experience of pain can feel all encompassing: the individual can at times be unable to look beyond his/her current experience of pain (Mossey & Gallagher 2004). It starts to define and colour all other experiences (Turk et al 1995).

Accordingly, the extant literature is clear in demonstrating the psychological and 'social' effects that pain can (and does) have on the individual. Moreover, each of the effects of pain listed in Box 4.2, to a greater or lesser extent, will either directly or indirectly lead to a greater sense of disconnection from humanity. An 'indirect' example, the inability to function and lethargy inevitably lead to less inclusion in social functions, interpersonal relationships and thus a greater sense of disconnection; whereas a 'direct' example would be having less interactions with one's friends. Thus, it becomes apparent that pain, be it physical or psychological in origin, has another effect on the person and that is to create or enhance the person's experiential sense of disconnection from humanity; although we have said 'be it physical or psychological in origin', it may be unhelpful to posit such simplistic 'Aristotelian' either/or depictions of pain as it is most likely to be 'and/both'.

So, to return to the notion of the cyclic nature of this relationship, in addition to pain leading to disconnection, we posit that the experiential sense of disconnection will, for some (if not many) be, in and of itself, a source of pain for the suicidal person. Theoretical evidence of this relationship already exists across a number of linked disciplines such as sociology, psychology, philosophy and nursing. We have already drawn attention to Durkheim's views on how pain (and ultimately suicide) can result from this sense of disconnection (lack of integration, alienation). The contemporary philosopher Sartre made similar remarks on the pain associated with an individual's sense of aloneness. Frankl (1959), Shneidman (1997), and Maris et al (2000) have drawn attention to the often difficult nature of life; under the best of conditions, life is often lonely and anxiety provoking and consequently a source of pain for the person (Maris 1982). Similarly, a large body of work exists within the domain of P/MH nursing which alludes to the need to be interpersonally connected. Regarded affectionately as 'the founding mother of psychiatric nursing', Peplau (1952, 1988) has repeatedly purported both the necessity of locating psychiatric nursing in an 'interpersonal' context and similarly, the therapeutic value of experiencing inter-personal connection – an empirical finding found repeatedly in studies that look at what people want and need from their mental health services. For example, in the study of Rogers et al (1993) on mental health service users' appreciation of psychiatric services in the UK (still the largest UK study of its kind), it was found that the preferred model of practice centred on involved personal contact. Related evidence from studies undertaken in numerous centres around the world affirms this interpersonal (and thus 'connected') form of P/MH nursing (see, for example, Avis et al 1994, Beech & Norman 1995, Cutcliffe et al 1997, Elbeck & Fecteau 1990, Gordon et al 1979, McIntyre et al 1989, Rudman 1996). More latterly, compelling findings reported in the Mental Health Foundation (2000) report 'Strategies for Living' once more reiterated the centrality of 'accepting relationships' and the value mental health service users place on such relationships.

Interestingly, there is another body of related work which speaks of disconnection and increased suicidality as it is experienced (and manifest) through the very basic human need of physical touch. Orbach's undeniable contributions in this area offer some illuminating evidence. Orbach (2003) summarizes his findings and reports results that point to suicidal youngsters having lower tactile sensitivity and responsiveness and lower emotional investment in the body. These suicidal youngsters were found to be disconnecting from the normal, required, basic human need of connection through touch and touching (see also Harlow & Soumi 1970). Related findings have been uncovered in associated areas, such as the empirical correlation reported between increased use of touch and physical comforting and survival rates in low-birth-weight infants (Feldman et al 2002, Sloan et al 1994).

Additionally, the French contemporary philosopher Gabriel Marcel (1948) constructed a persuasive and convincing argument about the nature of human existence and what he referred to as the 'ontological exigence'. According to Marcel, exigence refers to the person's need/demand for some level of coherence in the cosmos and more importantly (in terms of the issue of connectedness) for some understanding of one's place and role within this coherence. For Marcel, ontological *exigence* is not simply a wish or desire; it is not reducible to some psychological state, mood, or attitude. It is more central to existence than that; it is a movement of the human spirit that is inseparable from being human. To paraphrase, there is an alienable element of the human condition that is concerned with experiencing a sense of knowing one's place in the world; feeling connected to the world and others in it; feeling that one has a place and purpose. To live in the existential state then of feeling disconnected and to live with a pervasive sense of alienation, separateness, and isolation must be a dreadful source of psychological pain; of psychache.

THE PARTICIPANTS' EXPERIENCE OF DISCONNECTION: CONCEPTUALIZATIONS OF OUR DATA

The theoretical positions outlined above were echoed in the material provided by the participants in this study. The participants made reference to their existential position and subsequent experience while being in that suicidal 'place'. Participants spoke of how, prior to receiving any care/interventions from the suicide crisis teams, their overwhelming experiences were epitomized by feeling alone, isolated, hopeless, unsupported and withdrawn. Participants described how they felt misunderstood; felt that no one was listening to them. The participants explained how their sense of isolation was exacerbated as a result of being able to see only pain, further isolation (disconnection) and further hopelessness. Participants described how, when in their suicidal place, they felt they were a burden to their family and friends. This sense of being a burden sometimes extended to the healthcare system as well. The sense of been disconnected from humanity was further captured by the participants' statements about their feelings that everyone was against them, as a result, the participants no longer trusted humanity. Some referred to this disconnection in the form of their lack of functioning.

Importantly, some of the participants described this disconnection in the form of 'feeling dead already'; a nihilistic perspective. They spoke of feeling a sense of emptiness, nothingness, hopelessness, and pointlessness. Accordingly, as a result of analysis and conceptualization of the data, it became clear that the overwhelming existential state for the suicidal people in this study was one of feeling disconnected from humanity.

SOLVING THE KEY PSYCHOSOCIAL PROBLEM: RE-CONNECTING THE PERSON WITH HUMANITY

The key psychosocial process synonymous with care of the suicidal person is re-connecting the person with humanity. This is how the participants in the social setting resolved their key problem. In order to move the suicidal person from a 'death orientated' to a 'life orientated' position, it was necessary for the P/MH nurse to facilitate this re-connection with humanity. This re-connecting the person with humanity occurs over a three-stage process of healing, each stage having it's own conceptual heading, and these are described and explained in detail in the following chapters. The first stage is concerned with reflecting an image of humanity, and this appears to begin with a recognition that the person has indeed disconnected with humanity. This recognition can then set the 'tone' and the 'direction' of the intrapersonal and interpersonal work that needs to be done, namely – finding ways to re-connect the person with humanity and/or help the person gain a sense that he/she is indeed connected. The contact with the suicidal person at this stage needs to be intensive; the intensive contact which occurs in or at many levels, serves several purposes; not least it offers a direct contradiction to any experiences of lack of integration, social isolation and/or loneliness. The intensive contact is, in and of itself, both a tentative connection and a medium in which further connection can occur. It is important to point out that this intensive contact is purposeful, necessary and deliberate. Furthermore, this intensive contact should in no way be confused with the type of close physical proximity synonymous with defensive and custodial approaches to care of the suicidal person; most often expressed as 'close observations' or some synonym. (Where the practitioner engages only in close observations and follows the suicidal person around like some form of magnetic zombie; often saying nothing if anything to the person and having minimal interaction with the person.) This intensive contact also made possible the increased use of physical comforting and touch. Again, acknowledging as stated above, that suicidal people can even disconnect from this other form of basic human connection – touch, the healing potential of this was not lost on the P/MH nurses.

As the authors have noted earlier, suicide does not happen in a vacuum; fortunately the same can be said of care of the suicidal person. Indeed, the environment, both internal and external to the person, is used deliberately in a way to help facilitate the person's re-connection. As noted previously, suicide is often sought as a means to end one's psychache; a way of achieving peace from the sense of constant and pervasive pain. Thus, part of the facilitation of re-connecting the person with humanity involves helping the suicidal people find peace in other ways or through other means. The sense of peace then helps allow the person feel more connected.

Further, the sense of re-connecting with humanity is brought about in these early stages through re-establishing the person's trust in humanity. Through gaining trust in the nurse, the participant is then re-connecting with a person; taking the first tentative steps towards re-connecting with the wider community of 'humanity'. They achieved this through listening to and understanding the person; participants were very clear about how they often just needed someone to talk to during their 'recovery' from their suicide attempt and/or ideation. These interpersonal transactions and processes were not personified by erudite sentences or cleverly constructed deep analytical insights into the clients' psyche. The transactions were personified by the 'normalness' of the interactions and were most commonly described as 'just chatting'.

The key processes of communicating, being heard and understood, are some of the most basic, necessary and yet powerful interpersonal experiences; and yet simultaneously, eminently a human experience, perhaps one of the experiences that defines what it is to be human, to belong to the 'brother/sisterhood' of humankind (see Marcel's 1948 comments earlier in this chapter). In beginning, or re-commencing these communication processes, the participant can be seen to be entering into re-connecting with humanity. In the first instance, the person is re-connecting initially with the nurse who acts as a 'representative' of humanity. As stated above, the increasing sense of peace that arose from speaking and being listened to helped reduce the suicidal person's sense of psychache. The cathartic effect of talking through the situations and perceptions that had ushered the person towards suicide, and the 'novel' experience of finding someone whom is willing to listen without prejudice, are all immensely valuable processes in countering a person's sense of hopelessness and combating the person's desire to take their own life.

In addition, this re-connecting with humanity, brought about in this early stage by connecting first with the P/MH nurse, is brought about by the suicidal person increasingly feeling cared about and cared for; experiencing this sense and process of 'co-presencing'. Through demonstrating caring, compassion, and concern the P/MH nurse becomes the first 'point' of re-connection with humanity. The suicidal person connects with the nurse and thus begins to re-connect with humanity. This sense of being valued, feeling that they matter, helps the suicidal person realise that they are not alone, that their death would matter; that there are people around them who are invested in them as a human being. Further that there is immense therapeutic healing power in feeling cared about. It is a direct counter-action to the experiencing of 'psychache'.

As the process moves into its second stage, the re-connection with humanity was also brought about by experiencing the additional sense of security offered within the novel relationship, which allowed feelings, previously kept internalized by the person, to be discussed freely. It allowed the P/MH nurse to ask, 'Where does it hurt?' and allowed the suicidal person to respond. This externalization and subsequent rationalization of these thoughts permits the suicidal person to seek understanding of his/her feelings. There is appreciation that they do indeed need help. A connection is made between the internal turmoil and the fact that through talking with the P/MH nurse these feelings can be managed; that they can indeed discuss these thoughts and feelings without harming the P/MH nurse and therein would do no harm to their tenuous connection with humanity. Having previously felt controlled by their suicidal thoughts the suicidal person is able to take more responsibility over controlling *them*. The suicidal person also begins to re-connect with his/her pre-suicidal beliefs. During the times of high suicidality, the person's pre-suicidal beliefs, unfortunately, do not serve as strong enough protective factors; yet the original beliefs still have some protective value. Further, such beliefs were almost inevitably associated with feeling more connected with humanity. Building on the progress the suicidal person has begun to make connecting with humanity through connecting with the P/MH nurse and this connection is further strengthened by getting back in touch with these pre-suicidal beliefs. Now, with the additional support of their connection with the P/MH nurse, the suicidal person can once again draw on the protective elements contained within these beliefs.

Interestingly, despite being the *modus operandi* for some (many) practitioners and the primary treatment option, the use of medication had only a very limited part to play in this transformative process of recovery. The facilitative aspects were concerned with providing respite, albeit temporary respite, from the psychological pain and stress. More notably, the restrictive elements of the use of medication centred on increasing the person's sense of disconnection – most often as a result of the person feeling 'numbed, slowed down' and experiencing an altered level of mental functioning. This was especially the case if taking medication and meant that suicidal people were unable to resume their normal activities. It was also apparent when suicidal people themselves asked for and expected something more than medication and what they actually received was pharmacologically based 'help'. (Interestingly, the suicidal people in this study were adamant that they wanted the 'human touch' rather than 'more drugs'.) Additionally, part of the process at this stage involved attempts to re-frame constricted constructs through gentle challenge, offering alternative explanations and providing information. The constructs relating to a sense of disconnection, being different and worthless/hopeless are addressed and re-framed into essentially experiences that are the epitome of what it is to be human. Suicidal people are introduced to the constructs that what they are experiencing can very much be part of what it means to belong to the 'human community'; that their experiences are actually in keeping with others rather than being different. Further, that feeling disconnected is common and moreover, can be remedied.

This re-connection with humanity was also brought about as a result of the novel relationship between themselves and the nurse, and a product of this is that hope starts to emerge. While more work on promoting the re-emergence of hope appeared to occur in stage three, the beginnings of this re-emergence were evident in this stage. The person starts to look towards the future to see what it might hold for them. They move from questions of 'What happened to me?' to 'What *will* happen to me?' There is an increasing need to take control over their situation, where predominant in the early stage of the process the control of the situation was perhaps more with the P/MH nurse in their 'co-presencing' and guiding of the individual.

As the process moved into the third stage, this re-connection with humanity was brought about by the participant gaining understanding of, and beginning to make sense of his/her suicidality. In Stage 1, the P/MH nurse has offered a co-presence that has served to keep the suicidal person anchored to life, partly by reflecting an image of humanity. In Stage 2 the P/MH nurse provides information when asked, supporting the person emotionally and re-frames the suicidal person's negative constructs. In Stage 3 the continued presence of the P/MH nurse, albeit in different guises, represents a longitudinal re-connection; a thread that pulls the person back to the land of the living from the land of the dead, and offers a hand-hold on the path to the future. In other words, the P/MH nurse is the bridge that helps the suicidal person re-connect with humanity. The continuing professional presence of the P/MH nurse acts as a safety net, in case the process of re-connecting overwhelms the person and suicidality gains a foothold. The journey from death to life is an uphill struggle and the suicidal person needs emotional sustenance on the way. The support does not have to be physical, but may be virtual; knowing that there is a P/MH nurse who is a phone call away is sustaining in and of itself. However, this connectivity must be carefully managed. Its abrupt withdrawal may make the suicidal person feel that the P/MH nurse has lost interest in her/him and that attachment to the world of people and objects is not worthwhile.

This re-connection with humanity was also brought about by the suicidal person becoming more confident about the meaning of the suicide attempt and how it 'fits' into her/his past, present and future life trajectory. This understanding helps to give the suicidal person power over the suicidality, whereas before the suicidal person's sense of being and the suicidality were collapsed together. Putting the suicide in its place allows more space for re-connection. Consequently, it becomes possible to begin to make plans and set goals, which serve to help the suicidal person feel re-connected and hopeful. Without hope, the person can simply not be bothered to stay connected to her/his world. At this point, the P/MH nurse is continuing to be a resource, not undertaking the work for the suicidal person, but helping the person to project a positive future, encouraging the generation of ideas and possibilities.

This re-connection with humanity was also brought about by re-visiting the decision to commit suicide, considering whether life was, is and will be worth living. There is an acceptance by the suicidal person that she/he would have been missed (significant others may have expressed this directly) and this fuels the re-connection process. Further, by engaging in small, but significant, practical everyday activities the suicidal person begins to feel normal again, more a part of the human race; more connected. Success breeds success; as small changes occur, larger ones follow. Competency in the practical world is a barometer of hope.

CONCLUDING REMARKS

As with any other grounded theory, the findings captured in this chapter and explained in detail in the next three chapters, represent the most complete and robust theory of the way the participants solved their key psychosocial problem, at that time; however, the authors fully accept that this theory can (should?) evolve over time (Glaser 1992, Glaser & Strauss 1967). (Glaser's remarks indeed suggest that a grounded theory is never 'finished'.)

Accordingly, any new data uncovered in the future can be woven into the existing theoretical matrix and further delimit the categories and core variable.

Nevertheless, if this is a well constructed grounded theory it will fit the realities under study in the eyes of subjects, practitioners and researchers in the area and it will have 'conceptual grab'. Additionally, given that these are findings from a qualitative study, any attempt to infer nomothetic generalizable findings would be inappropriate and epistemologically flawed. The findings should, however, have idiographic (or naturalistic) generalizability; a generalizability about and based on the 'cases' (Sandelowski 1997). In this instance, the 'cases' were concerned with suicidal people who had received formal mental health care, principally from P/MH nurses. Thus, the findings should (can) have generalizability to other 'cases' involving formal care for suicidal people; irrespective of the similarities between different demographic groups (Denzin & Lincoln 1994). Research cases involving or focusing on the P/MH nursing care of the suicidal person should therefore bear a resemblance to care of the suicidal person as a 'whole' (Morse 1999). A process of caring identified in one setting, group or population can then be similarly experienced by another group (and have fit and grab for them too) or population in another setting.

With these thoughts in mind, the authors would like to draw attention to the latest view emanating from the WHO. In 2005, a consulting a group of suicidology experts including anthropologists, psychiatrists, sociologists, epidemiologists were brought together by the WHO and: 'They were unanimous in identifying a common denominator (in completed suicide cases) – a lack of connectedness. And this lack of connectedness permeates modern life, impacting society at three distinct levels – the family, the community, the workplace'.

The WHO's (2005) unequivocal response was to assert that: 'We have to revitalize our communities so that the connectedness people once felt in their communities, their workplaces and their families can be restored'.

The authors believe that the findings and theory described in this and the next three chapters contributes one part of the multi-dimensional and multi-professional theory that explains these much needed processes of re-connection in suicidal people.

Chapter 5

Reflecting an Image of Humanity – Stage One

'There were these two women sat on the edge of the bed dragging me back, mentally, intellectually and emotionally by making me engage with them.'
Interview N3

CHAPTER CONTENTS

INTRODUCTION

In this chapter we provide a detailed description and explanation of the specific qualities, interventions and activities that the P/MH nurse can use in order to provide meaningful care for the suicidal person. Recognizing that any process occurs over time and, according to Glaser (1978, 2001), will have at least two distinct phases or stages, this is the first of such stages and is one of the sub-core variables of our findings and subsequent theory. This stage was termed *'Reflecting an image of humanity'* and it captures the first stage of providing meaningful, therapeutic, transformative care for the suicidal individual.

We begin this chapter by providing an overview of the first stage and this is further illustrated by drawing heavily on direct quotes provided by the participants. We follow this with a more detailed explanation of the two key psychosocial processes (which represent the developed or de-limited theoretical categories) subsumed within this stage. These are termed: *'Experiencing intense, warm, care-based human-to-human contact'*, *'Implicitly challenging suicidal constructs as a result of encountering contrary experiences'*. Each of these is also explained and evidenced by drawing on direct quotes from the participants. In turn, these categories were developed and modified from six preliminary categories, therefore, we also describe, explain and substantiate each of these, and once again, support them with direct quotes. In order to help understand the construction and development of the findings, the developed and preliminary categories are listed in Boxes 5.1 and 5.2, respectively, and depicted in Figure 5.1. Accordingly, after reading this chapter, the practitioner should be more aware of the range of specific qualities, interventions and activities that the P/MH nurses used, and the suicidal people found to be of immense value and help. Further, the reader should be able to understand both the empirical background and theoretical development of these ways of working with suicidal people. As a result the findings should have more credibility, more spontaneous validity and more, to paraphrase Glaser (1978), fit and grab.

OVERVIEW

This sub-core variable is concerned with communicating a sense of care; communicating that the individual matters. For the participants in this study, having this sense that they mattered, that someone else was concerned about and interested in them, was immensely important and had a distinct countering effect on their suicidal ideation and perspectives. Feeling cared about created the perspective for the participant that he/she was no longer alone. The therapeutic value of such a sense or perspective in the context of providing care for the suicidal person should not be underestimated. The sense of being disconnected from humanity is directly countered by this connecting with the P/MH nurse. Participants in this study made clear references to the feelings that were stimulated when they experienced another person demonstrating an interest in their well-being. The participants were aware that they needed to feel that they mattered; they needed to feel that someone cared about them, and they were also very clear that they received such confirmation and validation from the P/MH nurses. The value of compassion, understanding and someone who was prepared to listen to them were also made clear by the participants. These 'fresh' and therapeutic experiences of feeling cared about, feeling that they mattered, feeling connected, all occurred in a very specific interpersonal atmosphere, one that was exemplified by the presence and influence of human warmth. Further, these experiences were directly opposite to their 'felt sense', namely, that they did not matter, that nobody cared about them, that it would not make a difference whether they lived or died. Additionally, it is important, although perhaps somewhat obvious, to point out that the presence of these qualities and feelings in the P/MH nurse (e.g. care and concern for the client's well-being, compassion, understanding) was not enough. The qualities and feelings also had to be communicated.

This sub-core variable is also concerned with facilitating the person's re-connection with humanity, and this is achieved in the first instance by connecting with the P/MH nurse. This re-connection with humanity is brought about by feeling cared about and cared for; experiencing this sense and process of 'co-presencing'. Through demonstrating caring, compassion and concern, the P/MH nurse becomes the first point of re-connection with humanity. The person connects with the P/MH nurse and thus begins to re-connect with humanity. In essence, this process shows how the P/MH nurse becomes a 'representative' or 'emissary' for humanity. When the person experiences this sense of being cared for by the P/MH nurse, they are at the same time, communicating that at least one 'part' of humanity still cares about the person. Engaging with the P/MH nurse in this way allows the participant to begin to internalize that they can still engage with humanity. The P/MH nurse's attitudes, demeanour and behaviour provide an 'in road', an opportunity to re-connect.

The data provided by the participants in this study indicate that suicidal people often need to have their basic needs met, including (if not especially) their fundamental need to feel connected to or engaged with other people. These basic needs are met by the P/MH nurse possessing (or adopting) and communicating: a sense of warmth for the person; care for the person; compassion for the person's situation and experience; a sense of hope and hopefulness for the person's future; unconditional acceptance and tolerance; empathy; understanding and positive regard. Further, in order to feel connected or re-connected with humanity, the person(s) needed to feel they could trust 'humanity'. Through developing a sense of trust in the P/MH nurse, the person is then re-connecting with another person; taking the first tentative steps towards re-connecting with the wider community of 'humanity'.

In addition, another key psychosocial process occurs in the first stage of this transformative recovery and that is the subtle, implicit challenge of the person's suicide constructs. Suicidal people experience the world and interpret the world in a very constricted and particular way and consequently form these distinctive suicidal constructs. The data provided by the participants indicted that P/MH nurses challenge these constructs essentially by means of what they are and what they do, and less by means of what they say. Throughout the interviews there was a clear sense of the participants' suicidal constructs; expressions of how they felt disconnected from humanity.

As a means to counteract these experiences and constructs the P/MH nurses would communicate and engage in a way that provided the 'opposite' experience. This subtle and gentle reflection provides the opportunity for suicidal people to consider some of their negative assumptions and challenge some of their restrictive beliefs. When the suicidal people in this study could begin to internalize that many of their beliefs about past failures, present limitations and future restrictions were based on unrealistic constructs and inaccurate self perceptions, they could begin to recognize that these constructs are perpetuated by their current state of hopelessness. Then they can begin to challenge these for themselves. As a result, the suicidal people in this study began to deconstruct some of their suicide constructs and hopelessness and began to construct a more hopeful future. The basic psychosocial processes of this sub-core variable were expressed and captured by the participants in the following ways:

'It is important that the nurses spent time with me; demonstrated that I was important; showed that I matter.' (Int. S2)

'They were a lovely mixture of professional but human.' (Int. N5)

'There were these two women sat on the edge of the bed dragging me back, mentally, intellectually and emotionally by making me engage with them.' (Int. N3)

'They are really good people and I like that. They were interested in me. I felt like I was in good hands.' (Int. N5)

'And then finally I had someone who understood how I was feeling.' (Int. S3)

'I was getting a lot of human warmth.' (Int. N5)

'I talked about what mattered in my life and he listened.' (Int. S3)

'It helped me not commit suicide, even though I was thinking about it, because I now knew there were people (the CAT – Community Assessment Team) who were bothered about me and didn't want me to.' (Int. N7)

'They (the CPNs – Community Psychiatric Nurses) would ask how I was feeling; he wanted to understand how I was feeling.' (Int. S3)

'The hour with the CPN. was a different experience to my usual experience of being completely locked into my own spiral of horror and death.' (Int. N3)

'I wanted someone to just talk to.' (Int. S2)

'I felt like the CAT team did care for me. They kept making sure that if I ever needed to speak to them I could just ring.' (Int. N7)

'It can only be good for people with an illness like mine to have someone come out and sit with them for an hour at a time; listening to my fears and just talking in general about whatever problems they may have.' (Int. S1)

'I felt that she was bothered about me; that I mattered to her.' (Int. N8)

'It was the regularity of them coming out and feeling like I was a priority.' (Int. S8)

'I could connect with Val because she came across as both a mum and a mate.' (Int. N8)

'It is marvellous when someone cares; to know that someone in that field (mental health care) knows what you are feeling.' (Int. S3)

'After talking to my nurse, instead of thinking 'Oh my God, I might as well kill myself', I was thinking, 'Right, what can I do to put this right'. (Int. N2)

'I didn't like talking to the psychiatrist who made notes as I was talking. (With the nurse) it was more open, more human, more natural, and more friendly.' (Int. S8)

'I was able to talk about the things that had been making me feel so low.' (Int. N2)

'My improvement had to do with the people and the talking.' (Int. S8)

'The nurses didn't come in with lectures and instructions, they came in to listen to me and that created trust.' (Int. N9)

'You just need the nurses to listen because you want them to be there to help you. They (the clients) might blurt out everything that is on their mind or they might sit for half and hour before they say anything because they don't have the strength to speak about it. So put everything in their control and say, 'Right, this is your floor, you take over and tell me, or if you don't want to speak I will just sit here with you, if you just want the company'. Just be there for them (the clients), be compassionate.' (Int. N5)

THE DEVELOPED CATEGORIES

> **Box 5.1 Reflecting an image of humanity (stage one): developed categories**
>
> - Experiencing intense, warm, care-based human-to-human contact
> - Implicitly challenging suicidal constructs as a result of encountering contrary experiences

Experiencing intense, warm, care-based human-to-human contact

Comparing new labels (new data) with existing labels and categories (existing data) enabled the preliminary categories (see below) to undergo further modification and integration. As a result, the category 'Experiencing intense, warm, care-based human to human contact' was induced. Integration and modification of certain preliminary categories (namely: *Intensifying contact, Building trust and familiarity, Talking about one's experiences and feeling understood, Communicating a sense of care that the individual matters*) indicated that each appeared to contain a similar process. One which suggested that this modified category is concerned with starting the process of re-connecting with humanity through connecting with the nurse. However, this connection with the P/MH nurse occurs as a result of the nurse's demeanour and attitude, the nurse's warmth towards the participant, the nurse's care and concern for the participant. In other words, the P/MH nurse unconditionally provides for the very basic and yet essential interpersonal needs. The value and importance of these most fundamental interpersonal processes was alluded to throughout the data. These common processes thus indicated the two properties of the category. Firstly, there is a property that is concerned with starting the process of re-connecting with humanity through connecting with the P/MH nurse. The second property is concerned with the attitudes, qualities and interventions that the P/MH nurse makes use of in order to facilitate this re-connection; it is a property that we refer to as 'co-presencing'.

Data provided by the participants, theoretical memos and the subsequent conceptualization of this material repeatedly indicated that participants made reference to how they would begin to connect with and thus feel comfortable with their P/MH nurse. These connections, at least in the beginning occurred at the most fundamental human level, gaining the existential experience that one is not alone. By talking, sometimes referred to as 'just chatting'; by laughing together; by both being there when the suicidal person experiences (and releases) any pent up pain. It may sound rather simplistic that the beginnings of recovery from their suicidal 'crisis' for these people in this study, were rooted in connecting with their P/MH nurse. On first consideration, it may appear too easy in that 'all' the P/MH nurse needs to focus on is demonstrating care, understanding and compassion. After all, that does not sound overly sophisticated or complex. However, within the theoretical and empirical suicide literature, there is a firm support for this finding. Suicidal people, probably as a result of a number of related factors, often feel disconnected from humanity, and often disconnected from themselves (see Orbach, 2003 for example). The need to feel connected to humanity; to have a sense of belonging, is a basic need (Aldefer 1972, Marcel 1948, Maslow 1962). Whether this is feeling connected to the *macro-level* of humanity or the *micro-level* (e.g. family, friends, colleagues), with the participants in this study, this basic need was not being met. Given the basic nature of the needs that are not being met, it should not be altogether surprising that 'basic' interpersonal 'interventions' are called for at this point in the process rather than anything more sophisticated.

This property explains the process of the P/MH nurse 'representing' or becoming an emissary for humanity. When the suicidal person experiences being cared for by a P/MH nurse, the nurse is communicating (perhaps implicitly) that humanity still cares about the person. Engaging with the P/MH nurse in this way allows the suicidal person to begin to internalize that they can still engage with humanity. The P/MH nurse's attitudes, demeanour and behaviour provides an 'in road', an opportunity to re-connect. Given the sense of disconnection to their loved ones that the participants described, it was unlikely that they would suddenly encounter a spontaneous re-connection with such people. Indeed, no such spontaneous re-connections were reported in this study. They needed P/MH nurses to facilitate this re-connection by being envoys. First enabling the suicidal person to internalize that they can engage and connect with the humanity in the form of the nurse, serves as the bedrock for future re-connection with the micro- and macro-levels of humanity. The processes within this property were described and captured by the participants in the following ways:

'I wanted to be with people who I knew cared about/loved me. I knew my nurse cared about me.' (Int. S1)

'I just needed someone to talk to as I had no support from anyone.' (Int. N2)

'I felt as though there was someone 'in there' with me; somebody caring for me.' (Int. S3)

'The nurse came on the Sunday and we just talked.' (Int. N3)

'It was easy to talk to my nurse because he respects me and I respect him, and that's why I like him so much.' (Int. S4)

'We would laugh together; if something was funny we laughed.' (Int. N5)

'Just to see a face, to tell them (the nurses) about my problem and feel that they understood it, was brilliant.' (Int. S4)

'I had been needing someone to talk to for a long time and couldn't get that from anywhere. So it was really good to finally have someone to talk to.' (Int. N2)

'It helped me so much to know that people (in this case the nurse) was thinking about me.' (Int. S8)

'I just wanted and needed someone to talk to as I felt so alone.' (Int. N5)

'I felt a bit better that someone had talked to me and realised that I needed help.' (Int. N7)

'It is very important that you have a cup of tea or something so that it isn't too professional.' (Int. N5)

'I don't know exactly what kind of help I do need, but I do know that I don't need someone patronizing me.' (Int. N8)

Data provided by the participants, theoretical memos and the subsequent conceptualization of this material repeatedly indicated how the P/MH nurses working with the participants possessed and communicated specific attitudes, qualities and demeanours. These qualities were the principal 'interventions' that the P/MH nurses made use of in order to facilitate this re-connection; they tried to reach a state of 'co-presencing', whereby the P/MH nurse was there, holistically, with the participant. Similarly, other 'interventions', such as they were, indicated that all interactions and engagements were personified by the atmosphere of warmth, care, compassion, unconditional acceptance and tolerance, empathy and positive regard for the participant. The therapeutic and healing power of these qualities has been shown repeatedly in the relevant empirical literature (see Adam et al 2003 for a further recent example). The participants in this study made reference to a lack of these qualities in their previous experiences. For some, these experiences had a direct influence on their increased risk (and subsequent attempt) of suicide. Consequently, it is not entirely surprising that the participants who had experienced a lack of these qualities gained such a beneficial, therapeutic effect from experiencing these qualities manifest in the P/MH nurse. Support for the therapeutic value of these qualities and attitudes is evident within the empirical suicide literature. Van de Wal's (1989) work offers a similar argument, though positing the value of these qualities as demonstrated and communicated by a mother or father to a child. He argues that as children identify with the mother and father's love for them, they internalize this for themselves; they learn to love and protect themselves. Similarly Anna Freud's (1949) theory posits that a warm, gentle, caring mother may tone down any (untamed) aggressive behaviours. There are clear parallels here with a P/MH nurse who can 'tone down' the suicidal person's self-focused aggressive behaviour, and can help the person to internalize their love and care for themselves (and thus give rise to self-protective rather than self-destructive behaviours) in response to the P/MH nurse's care, warmth, compassion, and 'love' for the suicidal person. The processes within this property were described and captured by the participants in the following ways:

'I had come to the conclusion that nobody cared. Thus what I needed was someone to convey that they did.' (Int. S1)

'My nurse was easy to communicate with. He could be quite funny (witty) at times, without laughing at me or my situation.' (Int. N2)

'The human warmth was crucial. They didn't just come in and get their stuff out. They looked me in the eye; they listened. Just chatting, even if it was going off at a tangent – was valuable. You know, when I said something, they didn't just move onto the next question.' (Int. N5)

'Q: What did the PET do? A: They listened.' (Int. S1)

'I remember having such freedom to talk.' (Int. N3)

'I got to release all my pent up emotion and grief over my granddaughter, with the C.P.N.' (Int. S3)

'He (C.P.N.) was a brilliant guy. He talked to me for an hour. The absolutely brilliant thing about it is there is no looking at clocks; no thinking you have only got ten minutes.' (Int. N5)

'I felt better for knowing that somebody could understand how I was feeling.' (Int. S3)

'I wanted and needed that 'human thing."' (Int. N5)

'They sat down and listened to me; showed me understanding when I cut my wrists.' (Int. S4)

'In terms of being the recipient of nursing, I would want a quick acceptance that what I am going through is a bit horrible.' (Int. N5)

'I felt understood and being understood was important.' (Int. S4)

'The difference with the nurses that helped me was the WAY they spoke to me.' (Int. N8)

'Frankie (nurse) was brilliant; she listened to everything I said.' (Int. S4)

Implicitly challenging suicidal constructs as a result of encountering contrary experiences

Comparing new labels (new data) with existing labels and categories (existing data) enabled the preliminary categories (see below) to undergo further modification and integration. As a result the category 'Implicitly challenging suicidal constructs as a result of encountering contrary experiences' was induced. Certain categories (namely: *Recognizing and acknowledging the antecedence and subsequent reality of the suicidal intent – disconnecting with humanity; Creating a relaxing internal and external environment; Building trust and familiarity; Talking about one's experiences and feeling understood; and Communicating a sense of care: that the individual matters*) indicated that each appeared to contain a similar process or processes to one another. These common processes thus indicated the three properties of the category. Firstly, there is a property that is concerned with the P/MH nurses recognizing that it is almost inevitable that people who are at high risk of suicide will have such suicidal constructs; these constructs may have been reinforced, but importantly, that they are still only constructs. Secondly, there is a property that is concerned with the P/MH nurses recognizing that too much explicit challenge early in the process of 'recovery' will only add to the sense of psychological pressure and thus they act accordingly; the challenge is left implicit. Thirdly, there is a property that is concerned with the P/MH nurses challenging these constructs essentially by means of what they are and what they do, in addition to what they say. The suicidal constructs of the client begin to be challenged by enabling the client to encounter these 'contrary' experiences.

Data provided by the participants, theoretical memos and the subsequent conceptualization of this material repeatedly indicated that these suicidal people often possessed a number of 'suicidal constructs'. The presence and influence of these constructs in the suicidal person is well documented in the associated literature. According to Beck et al (1990, p 190) a suicidal person can 'systematically misconstrue his or her experience in a negative way and anticipate dire outcomes to his or her problems'.

Schneider (1985) notes that 'the common cognitive state in suicide is constriction'. According to Schotte and Clum (1987), this constriction has also been described as cognitive rigidity and has been defined as a rigid style of perceiving and reacting to the environment that renders it difficult for a suicidal individual to formulate alternative approaches to problems. The suicidal person therefore experiences the world and interprets the world in a very constricted and particular way. Some of the origin of this constriction may be based in 'real' events and/or circumstances, e.g. experiencing stressful life events, living in poverty, living with unmet needs. Furthermore, these constructs may have been reinforced by certain life experiences and/or interactions with various people around the suicidal person (including some formal healthcare workers.) For example, one participant in this study spoke of how his feelings of worthlessness and disconnection from humanity were further exacerbated and 'reinforced' by the way he was 'treated' and dismissed by some formal healthcare individuals. Nevertheless, these constructs are still only that: constructs. They are interpretations of one's experiences; interpretations of one's place and value in the world; they are not necessarily 'truth'. Accordingly, as the participants in this study indicated, part of the role of the P/MH nurse is to acknowledge the reality of these thoughts and feelings for the suicidal person, yet at the same time, recognise them for what they are – interpretations of experience and subsequently, constructs. In this way the P/MH nurse communicates to the suicidal person that they are being heard, listened to and understood. The suicidal person begins to gain a sense that someone (finally) is listening and acknowledging the reality of the problem(s) as they are encountered and experienced by the person. The value and power of such actions on the part of the nurse was abundantly clear throughout the data in this study and clearly should not be underestimated. The processes within this property were captured and described by the participants in the following ways:

> 'I felt like my feelings were trivial.' (Int. S3)
> 'I felt as if everyone was against me. I couldn't trust my own family.' (Int. N1)
> 'When my mother died I felt like there was nothing what-so-ever. No point in going on.' (Int. N1)
> 'I felt like nobody wanted me so I might as well be dead.' (Int. N2)

Data provided by the participants, theoretical memos and the subsequent conceptualization of this material also repeatedly indicated that the suicidal people in this study often felt to be under an immense sense of psychological pressure. This sense of pressure only added to their increased risk of suicide. Our findings suggested that the P/MH nurses were very aware of this pressure and consequently, balanced the need to begin to challenge the individual's suicide constructs with the need to remove any sense of additional psychological pressure. Consequently, any such challenging of constructs was carried out implicitly (this is described in more detail below.) To begin to engage in challenge, especially overt challenge, so early in the process of recovery would only serve to exacerbate the individual's sense of pressure. At this stage in the process the suicidal people in this study needed to be free from having to solve problems; free from feeling the need to improve. While the suicidal people expressed a need to begin to re-connect with humanity, even this re-connection could not be forced or coerced; hence the need for a 'moment of pause', a time and space where the suicidal person can be free from the sense of having to strive. Thus to do anything other than reduce the sense of psychological pressure, particularly as a result of premature challenging, would only increase the risk of suicide. The processes within this property were described and captured by the participants in the following ways:

'I felt like nobody loved me. I came to the end of the line and wanted to kill myself. I felt like I couldn't fight it anymore.' (Int. S4)

'It's as though I was under a massive weight with everything bearing down on me.' (Int. N1)

'I was so ashamed of how I felt, I felt desperate, I just felt hopeless.' (Int. S3)

'I felt like I wasn't in control and it felt as if it was a dream.' (Int. N1)

Data provided by the participants, theoretical memos and the subsequent conceptualization of this material also repeatedly indicated perhaps the most important property of this category, namely, that P/MH nurses challenged these constructs essentially by means of what they are and what they do, and less by means of what they said. Throughout the interviews there was a clear sense of the participants' suicidal constructs; expressions of how they felt disconnected from humanity. As a means to counteract these experiences and constructs the P/MH nurses would communicate and engage in a way that provided an 'opposite' sense of the experience(s) and construct(s). This subtle and gentle reflection provided the opportunity for the suicidal people in this study to consider some of their negative assumptions and challenge some of their restrictive beliefs. When suicidal people can begin to internalize that many of their beliefs about past failures, present limitations and future restrictions are based on unrealistic constructs and inaccurate self perceptions and are perpetuated by their current state of hopelessness, then they begin to challenge these for themselves. The suicidal people begin to deconstruct some of their suicide constructs and hopelessness and begin to construct a more hopeful future.

For example, as participants spoke of their feelings and sense of hopelessness, the P/MH nurse would project hope and hopefulness into the atmosphere by remaining hopeful themselves. They brought hope with them into the interaction and this permeated into the 'emotional atmosphere' and was 'transplanted' into the participant by means of the close interpersonal connection (Cutcliffe 2004). The P/MH nurses would begin to introduce and articulate the possibility of hopeful outcomes. As the participants described how lonely they felt, the P/MH nurses would ensure that the suicidal people in this study were not alone. Not only in a physical sense, but they would communicate a sense that there was someone alongside them in their struggle. They would ensure messages of support, make sure there always being someone available for the suicidal person. The intensive, regular, warm and compassionate contact began to challenge, implicitly, the participants' construct of being alone. As the participants described how they felt that nobody cared about or loved them, the P/MH nurses would communicate how they cared very much about the total well being of the participant. How the participant's health, well being and future, mattered very much to the P/MH nurse. They would demonstrate that they were vested in the ongoing life of the participant.

Participants in this study also referred to the construct of having no-one to talk to. Here the P/MH nurses could provide a straightforward yet valuable intervention by offering themselves as someone to listen to the participant. Having had the experience of there being no-one with whom they could share their thoughts, feelings, fears and concerns, there was an immense sense of relief at finally being able to talk someone. Further, this experience served to challenge the construct that there is no-one to talk to. Bound up with this was the experience to counteract the participants' construct of feeling that their feelings are trivial. Throughout our interview data and findings is the clear evidence of the therapeutic power and value of the P/MH nurses 'being there' for the suicidal people in this study and validating them, their feelings/thoughts and experience. The fact that the P/MH nurses were more than willing to spend concentrated amounts of time focusing entirely on the participant's thoughts/feelings and experience provided a powerful challenge to the construct of 'my feelings are trivial'. They are direct and relevant responses to the expression of these feelings. There was also an exploration of what this must feel like for the participant.

When the suicidal people in this study described feeling ashamed, again the P/MH nurses counteracted this construct by demonstrating genuine acceptance, tolerance and communicate a sense of being non-judgemental; non-condemning. Again messages of support were common in response to such expressions and the P/MH nurses engaged in a lot of 'permission giving'. Informing the participants that thinking about or making an attempt on one's life need not be regarded as anything to be ashamed of; that such acts can be thought of as an expression of need. The processes within this property were described and captured by the participants in the following ways:

'I was able to get some of that need for companionship met by the PET.' (Int. S1)

'You feel that you are not alone because they (the nurses) are caring for you.' (Int. S3)

'It felt as though there were other people thinking about me and other people helping me.' (Int. S8)

'The CPN took an interest in what I was doing, what I did with my time, how I filled my days.' (Int. S3)

'They just changed my life, in just three days, because they were so loving and kind.' (Int. S7)

'I got a sense of being understood first of all by the person being there for me.' (Int. S3)

'The company, the presence of another who demonstrated care and concern, was crucial.' (Int. S4)

'The PET (Psychiatric Emergency Team) helped me by the support they gave, just support.' (Int. S4)

'The nurses communicated their care for me by means of – their sympathy, the expression on their faces, by means of the frequent phone calls.' (Int. S8)

'I was feeling that when they said that, they meant that. It wasn't just a trained response.' (Int. N5)

'What I got from the nurses was a bit of compassion; somebody to listen to me; a bit of understanding and somebody trying to help – and it did help.' (Int. N9)

THE PRELIMINARY CATEGORIES

> **Box 5.2 Reflecting an image of humanity (stage one): preliminary categories**
>
> J   Recognizing and acknowledging the antecedence and subsequent reality of the suicidal intent – disconnecting from humanity
> D   Intensifying contact
> B   Creating a relaxing internal and external environment
> E   Building trust and familiarity
> F   Talking about one's experiences and feeling understood
> H   Communicating a sense of care that the individual matters

Figure 5.1 Development of the stage one categories.

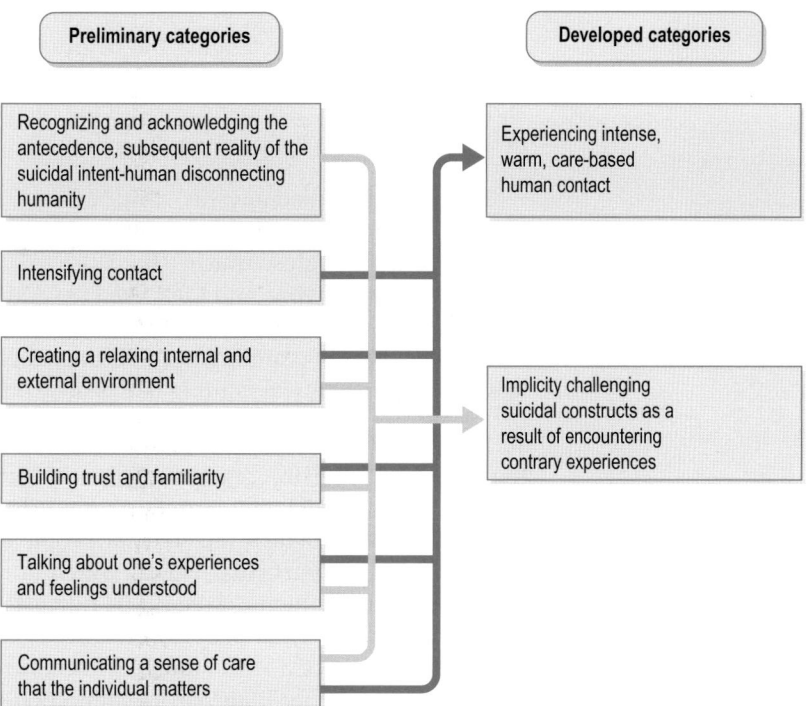

Preliminary category J: recognizing and acknowledging the disconnection with humanity and the reality of suicidal intent

The first preliminary category in this sub-core variable is concerned with *recognizing and acknowledging the antecedence and subsequent reality of the client's suicidal intent*. In essence, this category illustrates and explains the process wherein the P/MH nurse and suicidal person recognize that the person has become disconnected from humanity. The participants made reference to their existential position and subsequent experience while being in that suicidal 'place'. Participants spoke of their overwhelming experience of feeling alone, isolated, unsupported and withdrawn. The isolation they experienced as a result of being able to see only pain and further hopelessness. Participants described how, when in their suicidal place, they felt they were a burden to their family and friends. This sense of being a burden sometimes extended to the healthcare system as well. The sense of being disconnected from humanity was further captured by the participants' statements about their feelings that everyone was against them. Some referred to this disconnection in the form of their lack of functioning. Importantly, some participants described this disconnection in the form of feeling 'dead already'; a nihilistic perspective. They spoke of feeling a sense of emptiness, nothingness, hopelessness, and pointlessness. Within this process, it was important that the P/MH nurse recognized and accepted the validity of these perspectives and constructs. The experiences were not 'played down' or diminished to have no meaning; the description and narratives of the experiences were listened to; they were acknowledged and they were empathized with.

This category contains at least two properties. The first property is concerned with the suicidal people describing their experiences when in their suicidal place; describing in what particular ways they have disconnected with humanity; acknowledging the reality of their suicidal intent. The second property is concerned with the P/MH nurse hearing and accepting this, and simultaneously gaining a sense of the clients' particular needs. This was described by the participants in the following ways:

'I felt like I had died anyway.' (Int. N2)

'I didn't want to burden my family with my problems because they had already gone through so much.' (Int. S3)

'I didn't have anyone and I felt like I needed the support.' (Int. S2)

'When you are in the middle of pain, you can't see beyond it.' (Int. S8)

'So I knew I was planning it. I told the people I was seeing, I even dared to say that I knew it was coming to a head.' (Int. N8)

To conceptualize the key processes in this preliminary category, they are those of describing the disconnection with humanity and acknowledging the reality of the suicidal intent. Furthermore, the process of identifying the particular ways in which the suicidal people feel disconnected serves as a means to identify particular needs, which in turn, provides a preliminary focus to the interventions of the P/MH nurse. For example, and most importantly, when the suicidal people in this study began to verbalize their sense of feeling disconnected with humanity, then there was a clear requirement for the P/MH nurse to facilitate this re-connection. Additionally, there are more specific or finite forms in which this disconnection is expressed. For example, when the suicidal people spoke of feeling alone, feeling unsupported and feeling that nobody cares, then there are straightforward attitudes, demeanours, behaviours and interventions that the P/MH nurse can use to counter such perceptions and constructs.

Preliminary category D: intensifying contact

The next category in this sub-core variable is concerned with *intensifying contact*; intensifying the contact between the P/MH nurse and the suicidal person. In essence, this category illustrates and explains the process where the P/MH nurse ensures the person is seen on a frequent basis. The frequency was variable for different people, but it was always intensive and likely to be more frequent than for clients who are not in such a crisis. Furthermore, occasionally the contact was constant and for 24 hours a day. The participants in this study described how valuable such intensive and frequent contact was. They described this regular contact as something that they looked forward to, even though at first it was occasionally experienced as intrusive and intimidating. The participants also alluded to the proportionate relationship that appears to exist for some between suicidal ideation/risk and the need for more intensive/frequent contact.

This category contains at least two properties. The first property is concerned with the frequency of contact; whether this is on a moment by moment basis, a day to day basis or a week by week basis. The second property is concerned with how the suicidal people in this study experienced this contact and how these experiences were not static but were fluid. This was described by the participants in the following ways:

'When I was feeling really suicidal, that's when I needed the most companionship.' (Int. S1)

'Just as long as I knew they were coming (every two days), I knew he would be there and we could go out.' (Int. S8)

'I needed that duration of time and input at that time.' (Int. N2)

'I saw the CAT daily in the beginning.' (Int. N3)

To conceptualize the key processes in this category, they are those of creating a sense of closeness, both emotionally and physically. The suicidal people in this study verbalized their sense of being disconnected from humanity, and at the same time, some referred to the need to feel close to humanity. The intensive contact provided by the nurses in this study is far more than the somewhat 'crude', defensive and unsophisticated 'close observations'. The suicidal people in this study were 'reaching out' for human contact, human closeness and the P/MH nurses recognized and responded to this need. Also there is the process of keeping the person physically safe. It would be naïve not to recognize that the intensive contact does include a property of maintaining the suicidal client's safety. Nevertheless, most often, this was a subsidiary process to the more predominant process of providing human closeness. For example, realistically, how much physical safety is provided by a P/MH nurse who sees the client for 1 hour out of the 24 hours in a day? However, the knowledge that 'their' P/MH nurse was coming to see the suicidal person did provide them with a sense of safety and thus, this process needs to be acknowledged.

Preliminary category B: creating a relaxing internal and external environment

The next preliminary category in this (sub) core variable is concerned with *creating a relaxing internal and external environment*. The participants made reference to how there were specific efforts made by the P/MH nurses to remove any sense of psychological pressure and how this was exactly what they needed at that time. The P/MH nurses modelled calmness; had calmness about them; communicated to the suicidal person that there is no sense or hurry or rush. There was a sense of allowing the person to be introspective, if, at that time, that's what they needed to be. There was a sense of not adding to the suicidal person's sense of psychological psychache and pressure by making the person feel they had to behave in a certain way. There was no urgency to explain why the person was feeling suicidal. Furthermore, for some of the suicidal people in this study, the formal care teams would temporarily take control for a while if needs be. This was manifest in many ways, including: taking care of day-to-day tasks for the person; contacting various agencies; and making sure the person's support systems were activated. It is important to note that any control taken on by the P/MH nurses was temporary and carried out if the person was feeling overwhelmed by having to tend to the various issues. In addition to these, there was also a process of creating the healthy, pressure-free environment by encouraging the suicidal person to be in the physical environment where they felt most relaxed. Interestingly, many of the suicidal people in this study opted to be cared for at home because they felt less pressure there. However, some of the participants did want to be 'away from it all' and felt hospital admission would give them this sense. The P/MH nurses also provided specific relaxation sessions and taught relaxation techniques, both of which were experienced as extremely beneficial by the suicidal people.

This category contains at least two properties. The first property is concerned with the P/MH nurses facilitating and nurturing the appropriate internal or 'individual psychological' environment where the suicidal person felt most free from pressure and stress. The second property is concerned with P/MH nurses structuring and placing the suicidal people in the most appropriate physical environment where they felt most free from pressure and stress. This was expressed by the participants in the following ways:

'The absence of pressure and the sense of calm were very important to me.' (Int. N1)

'The team was always calming and re-assuring.' (Int. S1)

'You need to be cared for at home, in your own environment, in a familiar and relaxed environment.' (Int. S1)

'I can remember that the most important thing for me was to relax because I was feeling so pent up. And the relaxation really helped. (It gave me)..such a good feeling; a sense of inner peace.' (Int. S3)

'When the C.A.T. came to see me they were quite calm with me. They made sure that it was going to be a relaxed atmosphere.' (Int. N7)

To conceptualize the key processes in this category, there are two distinct though linked processes occurring. Firstly, is the process of creating and/or facilitating the sense of freedom from the 'psychache'. In the knowledge that stress and 'psychache' are clear contributors to a person's risk of suicide, the P/MH nurses remove all the stress they can. In removing or reducing the suicidal person's sense of stress, the risk of suicide is thus diminished. The second process goes to the peace and calmness created, which communicated a sense to the suicidal person that the expected sense of peace and relief from psychological pain, that they assume will only come from death, can be achieved without killing themselves. Accordingly, the beginnings of the change in the cognitive processes within the suicidal person that need to occur (the shift from hopelessness to hope), is stimulated. As the suicidal people in this study began to internalize their new experience, namely that the only option for peace and calmness is not death, they began to challenge their suicidal orientated construct; namely, that death is the only viable option.

Preliminary category E: building trust and familiarity

The next category in this sub-core variable is concerned with *building trust and familiarity*; trust and familiarity between the suicidal person and the P/MH nurse. The category is concerned with building a therapeutic closeness and firm interpersonal connection between the suicidal person and P/MH nurse. This relationship is located in a 'professional' context, yet is most often manifesting as a form of 'friendship'. As a result the suicidal people in this study referred to the development of a 'professional friendship.' Importantly, the presence of both contexts was necessary; the one without the other did not provide the suicidal people with what they needed. The 'natural' or 'normalness' of the P/MH nurse and the nurse's interactions was clear and indeed, welcomed by the participants. However, at the same time, the P/MH nurse's professional experience and competence was a source of comfort and helped the development of trust. The suicidal people in this study were very clear that they needed to believe in their P/MH nurse. Furthermore, participants referred to the importance of the sense of mutual respect that needed to be present. This was often manifesting in the form of treating the suicidal person like an adult; an individual; not 'talking down' to them. The participants also spoke of the other processes involved in creating and developing a sense of trust, including the value of listening; genuinely listening to the person. The use of carefully timed and appropriate humour was also described. While, on initial consideration, it may appear incongruous and potentially insulting to use humour at such sensitive times, the use of humour helped build trust, create a sense of normalness; a sense of familiarity. Lastly, and crucially, much of the sense of trust and familiarity was achieved by, not so much what the P/MH nurse did or said, but by the way they said it. The P/MH nurse's demeanour and attitude were described as being vital to the development of trust and familiarity. This demeanour was, again, personified by demonstrating humanness, warmth, understanding, empathy, approachability, a nonjudgemental attitude, and care.

This category contains at least two properties. The first property is concerned with the value and importance ascribed by the participants to feeling that they could trust the P/MH nurse. The second property is concerned with the actual processes of forming and building trust. This was described by the participants in the following ways:

'It is important that trust is there in the relationship. I would say about 95% of it is trust.' (Int. S1)

'It is like we are mates.' (Int. S4)

'The humor helped at times.' (Int. N2)

'Simple things made me feel better; the nurse's attitude, his manner, his demeanour.' (Int. S4)

'The Community Psychiatric Nurse (CPN) was persistent and trustworthy and this enabled my trust to build; which led to a breakthrough.' (Int. N3)

To conceptualize the key processes in this category, there are important processes here that are clearly part of the 'larger' processes of re-connecting with humanity. The establishment and maintenance of trust is not something that occurs instantly; it is a process that needs to be worked at; it can develop over time. Nevertheless, in order for the trust process to flourish, the appropriate and facilitative attitudes and demeanours needed to be present from the first moment of contact. In order to feel connected or re-connected with humanity, the participants needed to feel they could trust 'humanity'. Through gaining trust in the P/MH nurse, the participant is then re-connecting with a person; taking the first tentative steps towards re-connecting with the wider community of 'humanity'. In addition to this, in gradually re-connecting with the P/MH nurse, the suicidal people in this study learned again that they are capable of re-connecting with humanity; with the lived. Their constructs and sense of isolation and disconnection are then challenged.

Preliminary category F: talking about one's experiences and feeling understood

The next category in this (sub) core variable is concerned with the suicidal people *talking about their experiences and feeling understood*; understood by their P/MH nurse. Throughout the interviews the participants referred to how they felt the need to be understood. The participants were adamant that they needed to feel that someone understood their experience and their plight. Additionally, when they felt they were being listened to and understood, this had a profound therapeutic effect on them. Participants were very clear about how they often just needed someone to talk to during their 'recovery' from their suicide attempt and/or ideation. The importance and value of listening to the suicidal people in this study was not lost on the P/MH nurses. Participants described how the P/MH nurses would make specific attempts to listen and communicate that they wanted to understand. They were interested in the suicidal people, in their stories, in their experiences and heard these narratives without passing judgement or condemning the person's behaviour.

In addition, the participants explained how in talking about their experiences and gaining a sense that they were being understood, they encountered a cathartic release, a feeling of emancipation and liberation. They were somehow 'lighter' emotionally having had this catharsis; their sense of psychache was lessened. It was also of particular note that these interpersonal transactions were not personified by erudite sentences, cleverly constructed deep analytical insights into the suicidal person's psyche. The transactions were personified by the 'normalness' of the interactions; and was most commonly described as 'just chatting'. As a result of the talking, hearing, being listened to and feeling understood, the participants also gained a sense of feeling less isolated, less alone. They began to experience this sense of re-connecting with another person. Some of the suicidal people in this study described another therapeutic process (or outcome) of talking about their experiences and feeling understood. The effect of this experience was to counter or combat their previous experiences of not being listened to. Whereas in the past, these people had wanted to talk and wanted to feel listened to, they had not received this and one result of this was the growth of their suicidal ideation (and resultant increase in risk). Consequently, their experience within this therapeutic relationship was directly what they needed in order to begin to reduce their suicide ideation and related risk.

This category contains at least four properties. The first property is concerned with the suicidal person's need to feel heard, listened to and understood. The second property is concerned with the immense therapeutic value of 'just talking'. The third property is concerned with the skills that the P/MH nurses used to hear and listen to people and at the same time, communicate a sense that they were hearing. The fourth property is concerned with how this experience of being heard and understood countered the previous prohibitive and constricting experiences that some suicidal clients in this study had. This was described and captured by the participants in the following ways:

'It is very important to feel that someone understands what I am feeling.' (Int. S3)

'Talking to the nurses helped me, that made me feel better, that helped.' (Int. S1)

'I had been feeling so insecure, but having someone to talk to provided me with a bit of security.' (Int. N2)

'The team helped me by listening to me, trying to understand my problems at the time.' (Int. S4)

'It was very supportive to spend two or three hours with someone just chatting.' (Int. S2)

'I found it was more re-assuring that at least somebody was going to listen to me now and offer me some help of some sort.' (Int. N2)

'The CAT didn't judge me when I spoke; they made me feel that they were there to help me.' (Int. N7)

'I knew I was being listened to when they answered me, gave me answers I could relate to.' (Int. S8)

'The way my nurse listened, the way he was so attentive, made a difference, set him apart from other professionals who didn't really help me much in the past.' (Int. N2)

To conceptualize the key processes in this category, as with the preliminary category: *communicating a sense of care, that the individual matters*, the key processes are those of the beginnings of re-connecting with humanity. The key processes of communicating, being heard and understood, are some of the most basic, necessary and yet powerful interpersonal experiences. In so beginning, or re-commencing these communication processes, the suicidal person can be seen to be re-connecting with humanity. In the first instance, perhaps re-connecting with the P/MH nurse, who acts as a 'representative' of humanity. At the same time as this re-connection occurs there is the immense therapeutic value in the process and experience of talking about one's experiences and being listened to and understood. The 'off loading' of the stress as one talks about the trials and tribulations of life, the cathartic effect of talking through the situations and perceptions that had ushered the person towards suicide and the 'novel' experience of finding someone whom is willing to listen without prejudice, are all immensely valuable processes in countering a suicidal person's sense of hopelessness and psychache, and combating the suicidal person's desire to take his/her own life.

Preliminary category H: communicating a sense of care; that the individual matters

The next category in this sub-core variable is concerned with *communicating a sense of care*; communicating that *the individual matters*. For the participants in this study, having this sense that they mattered, that someone else was concerned about and interested in them was immensely important and had a distinct countering effect on their suicidal ideation and perspectives. Feeling cared about created the perspective for the participant that he/she was no longer alone. The therapeutic value of such a sense or perspective in the context of providing care for the suicidal person should not be underestimated. The sense of being disconnected from humanity was directly countered by this connecting with the P/MH nurse. Participants in this study made clear references to the feelings that were stimulated when they experienced the interest in their well-being from another person. The participants were aware that they needed to feel that they mattered; they needed to feel that someone cared about them, and they were also very clear that they received such confirmation and validation from the P/MH nurses. The value of compassion, understanding and someone who was prepared to listen to them was also made clear by the participants. These 'fresh' and therapeutic experiences of feeling cared about, feeling that they mattered, feeling connected, all occurred in a very specific interpersonal atmosphere; one that was exemplified by the presence and influence of human warmth. Additionally, it is important, although perhaps somewhat obvious, to point out that the presence of these qualities and feelings in the P/MH nurse (e.g. care and concern for the client's well-being, compassion, understanding) was not enough. The qualities and feelings also had to be communicated.

This category contains at least two properties. The first property is concerned with the suicidal person's sense of being valued and the immense therapeutic effect that this had on them. The second property is concerned with the ways and methods that the P/MH nurses used to communicate a sense of these qualities and feelings. Perhaps this second property is captured by the concept/process of 'co-presencing': the process of being with a person and communicating, often in very subtle ways, that the person matters, that the P/MH nurse cares about the well-being of the suicidal person, that the suicidal person gets the sense that the P/MH nurse is concerned about them as a human being. This was expressed by the participants in the following ways:

'I had come to the conclusion that nobody cared. So what I needed was a sense that somebody did (and this was provided by the PET.' (Int. S1)

'It was important that the nurses spent time with me; demonstrated that I was important; showed that I mattered.' (Int. S2)

'They (the PET) were bothered about me, and it was very important to feel that they are bothered about me.' (Int. S3)

'As a result of being contacted I thought, 'At least somebody is looking and acting as if they care about me' and I thought that was really nice.' (Int. N2)

'My nurse was not pushy, and that' was what I needed at the time. Not to be pushed, but to feel that he was bothered about me.' (Int. N1)

'Yes, it was very helpful for me to know that they (the CAT) were thinking about me; that they were there; that they are concerned about me; that they have an understanding of what I am going through.' (Int. S8)

To conceptualize the key processes in this category, it should be noted that there are important processes occurring. As with the preliminary category 'Building trust and familiarity', these processes are pivotal to and preliminary in the overall process of re-connecting with humanity. This re-connection with humanity is manifest through the connection with the P/MH nurse, which is brought about by feeling cared about and cared for; experiencing this sense and process of 'co-presencing'. Through demonstrating caring, compassion, and concern the P/MH nurse becomes the first 'point' of re-connection with humanity. The suicidal person connects with the P/MH nurse and thus begins to re-connect with humanity. Furthermore, there is an important, though implicit process and that is the challenge to the person's suicidal constructs that experiencing these genuine expressions of care brings about. This sense of being valued, feeling that they matter, helps the person realise that they are not alone, that their death would matter, that there are people around them who are invested in them as a human being. Further that there is immense therapeutic healing power in feeling cared about; for the participants in this study, it was a direct counter-action to the experiencing of psychache.

Chapter 6

Guiding the Individual Back Towards Humanity – Stage Two

'Putting my life into a different perspective – seeing things in a different, more positive way, really made a difference and it was my time with my nurse and the CAT team that did that.'
Interview N2

CHAPTER CONTENTS

INTRODUCTION

In this chapter we provide a detailed further description and additional explanation of the specific qualities, interventions and activities that the P/MH nurse can use in order to provide meaningful care for the suicidal person in this stage of the process. Recognizing that any process occurs over time and, according to Glaser (1978, 2001), will have at least two distinct phases or stages, this is the second of such and is one of the sub-core variables of our findings and subsequent theory. This stage was termed *'Guiding the individual back towards humanity'* and it captures the second phase of providing meaningful, therapeutic, transformative care for the suicidal individual.

We begin this chapter by providing an overview of the second stage and this is further illustrated by drawing heavily on direct quotes provided by the participants. We follow this with a more detailed explanation of the three key psychosocial processes (which represent the developed or de-limited theoretical categories) subsumed within this stage. These are termed: *'Nurturing insight and understanding'*, *'Supporting and strengthening pre-suicide beliefs'* and *'Encouraging a novel interpersonal, helping relationship'*. Each of these is also explained and evidenced by drawing on direct quotes from the participants. In turn, these categories were developed and modified from six preliminary categories, therefore, we also describe, explain and substantiate each of these, and once again, support them with direct quotes. In order to help understand the construction and development of the findings, the developed and preliminary categories are listed in Boxes 6.1 and 6.2, respectively, and depicted in Figure 6.1. Accordingly, after reading this chapter, the practitioner should be more aware of the range of specific qualities, interventions and activities that the P/MH nurses used in stage two, and the suicidal people found to be of immense value and help. Further, the reader should be able to understand both the empirical background and theoretical development of these ways of working with suicidal people. As a result the findings should have more credibility, more spontaneous validity and more, to paraphrase Glaser (1978), fit and grab.

OVERVIEW

'Guiding the individual back towards humanity' signals the arrival of a new stage in the person's ability to make a connection with the world about them. In stage one the person gains a sense of re-connection with humanity through the act of being cared about and 'co-presencing'. This relationship, built up between the P/MH nurse and the suicidal person, now takes on a different pace. During this stage there is a more active focus to this process of reconnection, whereas previously, in stage one, the clear focus for the P/MH nurse was on 'being' rather than 'doing'. Concerned as they were, with guiding the person back to humanity, in this second stage the P/MH nurses attempted to nurture insight and understanding; particularly a renewed insight and understanding *vis a vis* control. The participants in this study were very clear that an increased sense of control *over* their suicidal thoughts and feelings rather than the suicidal thoughts and feelings having control *over them*, was not only extremely important but further, it was indicative of re-connecting with

humanity. In gaining or re-gaining insight into and understanding of their experiences and situation, not least in part by reconstructing or reframing certain constricted personal constructs, the suicidal people begin to see that they are not as irremediably disconnected from humanity as they once thought; there is still a way back. Furthermore, the increased insight and understanding was concerned with a new awareness of the suicidal person's increased need for help; in some cases a recognition that they needed to reach out to humanity, reach out to the P/MH nurse as a means of helping the person overcome their suicidal ideation.

The data provided by the participants indicated that suicidal people often feel they are a burden to those family and friends who are close to them. It is not until the P/MH nurse has a strong bond that the suicidal people in this study were able to express their emotions to their nurse; and the unburdening of problems with the P/MH nurse indicates that a re-connection with humanity is present. Prior to this stage, withdrawal and disconnection had interfered with and inhibited communication. The seeds of hope and hopefulness projected by the P/MH nurse in stage one are then nurtured by the nurse in this stage and start to re-surface in the individual. This hope is drawn out and strengthened by the P/MH nurse's attention to the suicidal person's positive attributes and the nurse's complete faith in the person's ability to deal with their problems, given the appropriate help and support. The P/MH nurse encouraged the suicidal people in this study to use their own belief systems to enhance this process and, as a result, the people started to move towards a 'life position' rather than opting for suicide. By opening up the communication between P/MH nurse and suicidal person, a more active, therapeutic basis to the relationship is encouraged. The suicidal people were more accepting of the tools offered to them by the P/MH nurse. In turn the suicidal people in this study started to ask for explanations for the way they were feeling. Although progressing from stage one, the suicidal person is not comfortable being left without support. Support comes from human contact, from the P/MH nurse and/or the suicidal person's significant others. The psychosocial processes within this sub-core variable are exemplified within the study participants' own words.

'The nurses gave me a positive attitude as I hadn't always felt positive'. (Int. S3)

'They let me come out of myself and talk more frankly than I would to other people'. (Int. N3)

'They changed the way I was viewing the world. This has made a big difference. It made me stop and start to think again – more positively'. (Int. S1)

'I could say what I wanted to my nurse, even things about my feelings and I have difficulty with that, even with my wife'. (Int. N1)

'I thought to myself – I'm going to fight this'. (Int. S3)

'The more I talked, the more understanding of my conflict I gained and the less likely I was to get into my downward, deep spiral'. (Int. N3)

'It was so helpful in being able to recognize that I had an internal conflict going, and through talking about it I could identify what was going on for me'. (Int. N3)

'They gave me handouts/information on the signs and symptoms of anxiety'. (Int. S3)

'. . . coping strategies, some tools; I think that was important. When I first went to the services what I needed from people were tools'. (Int. N5)

'It was important and helpful to be able to talk about my problems with my nurse, and feel that they understood me, because I don't get this anywhere else not even from my family'. (Int. S4)

'It was encouraging to know that the CAT team thought I was strong enough to get through this'. (Int. N7)

'We talked about what I thought were the positive things in my life. It was good not to just focus on the bad'. (Int. N7)

THE DEVELOPED CATEGORIES

> **Box 6.1 Guiding the Individual back to humanity (stage two): developed categories**
>
> - Nurturing insight and understanding
> - Supporting and strengthening pre-suicidal beliefs
> - Encountering a novel interpersonal, helping relationship

Nurturing insight and understanding

Comparing new labels (new data) with existing labels and categories (existing data) enabled the preliminary categories (see below) to undergo further modification and integration. As a result two new developed categories were induced and another was further developed, though it still retained its original name. The first of these is *nurturing insight and understanding*. Certain preliminary categories (namely: *having personal awareness of Gestalts and moments of insight, recognizing the limit and value of pharmacological intervention, and teaching and explaining*) indicated that each appeared to contain a similar process or processes to one another, and these common processes thus indicated the three properties of the category. Predominantly the key process is concerned with facilitating the rise in the suicidal person's personal awareness and having the ability to subsequently externalize these moments of awareness. A connection is made between the internal turmoil and the fact that, through talking with the P/MH nurse, these feelings can be managed. Having previously felt controlled by their suicidal thoughts the suicidal person is able to take more responsibility over controlling *them*. Furthermore, it is important to note another important shift from phase one to phase two. Each of the developed categories in this core variable indicate a more active focus to this processes, whereas previously in stage one, the clear focus was on 'being' rather than 'doing'.

Nurturing insight and understanding contains at least three properties. The first of these relates to the suicidal person's ability to make a link between internal feelings and the subsequent actions. It relates to a growth in awareness that the suicidal person *can* have power over these thoughts and feelings; that they do not necessarily have to expect a dire future; an awareness that a hopeful future is a possibility. The second property relates to a rise in the suicidal person's awareness of what type(s) of help needed, and perhaps more importantly, what they found to be helpful and unhelpful.

A further aspect of this property refers to the suicidal person's increasing willingness and ability to articulate what they need from their P/MH nurse and from the formal mental healthcare system. It is noteworthy that the suicidal people were adamant and vociferous about articulating what they did not want. Of special importance, particularly in terms of the current *modus operandi* for care of the suicidal person, and the current emphasis within this approach, are the suicidal people's remarks about the limitations and value of pharmacological intervention. We return to this important aspect in Chapters 8 and 9. The third property relates to the suicidal person's readiness to accept the help offered to them by the P/MH nurse.

The authors have already pointed out, in Chapter 5, that suicidal people can systematically misconstrue their experience(s), and invariably anticipate dire outcomes to their problems, including the outcome of their own future (Beck et al 1990, Schneider 1985, Weishaar 2000). Data provided by the participants, theoretical memos and the subsequent conceptualization of the material obtained in this present study, repeatedly indicated that one such constricted construct that the suicidal people often possessed was a sense of inevitable doom; a lack of control related to a hopeless future. There is an established, though relatively underdeveloped literature that refers to what is sometimes termed 'dysfunctional assumptions' (Beck et al 1990, Bonner & Rich 1987, Ellis & Ratliff 1986, Raneiri et al 1987, Weishaar 2000). Ellis and Ratliff (1986) reported how suicidal psychiatric inpatients scored higher than non-suicidal patients in terms of various dysfunctional assumptions. Very similar findings are reported by Bonner and Rich (1987) who discovered that these dysfunctional assumptions are a key indicator in predicting suicidal ideation in college students. Raneiri et al (1987) also found a positive correlation between severity of dysfunctional assumptions and suicidal ideation in psychiatric inpatients. As a result, if we accept these consistently reported findings as credible, it seems that one possible method of, at least in part, combating a person's risk of suicide is to attempt to address these dysfunctional assumptions. Accordingly, the findings reported in this might not be considered surprising; a growth in awareness in the suicidal person that he/she has dysfunctional assumptions helps the suicidal person move back towards a 'life orientated' stance. These properties are expressed and captured in the participants' own words:

'It was so helpful in being able to recognize that I had an internal conflict going on, and through talking about it I could identify what was going on for me'. (Int. N3)

'It was the encouragement and the reminder that I had some control, some responsibility – that I could help myself'. (Int. S8)

'I intended to get better and realised that I had an opportunity – what with the kindness and people similar to me'. (Int. S3)

'I was ready to accept help when it was offered'. (Int. N2)

'Talking about my son and what I could have done to him had a big effect on me not taking my life'. (Int. N1)

'The more I talked the more understanding of my conflict I gained and the less likely I was to get into my downward, deep spiral'. (Int. N3)

'They gave me handouts on the signs and symptoms of anxiety'. (Int. S3)

'They explained things to me'. (Int. S4)

'. . . what I wanted from people were some tools'. (Int. N5)

'I saw the doctor and he put me on some anti-depressants, but I said to him that I really needed some counselling'. (Int. N2)

'I felt more in control after my medication'. (Int. S4)

'They changed my medication and I felt brilliant'. (Int. S1)

'I would not have got better if all I had received was more tablets'. (Int. S3)

'The tablets did me some good in that they calmed me down'. (Int. S1)

'The doctors prescribed me some Peroxatine, and I started to take those, but the side effects kicked in bad enough for me not to be able to go to work'. (Int. N5)

Supporting and strengthening pre-suicidal beliefs

Through a process of modification of the preliminary categories the new developed category 'Supporting and strengthening pre-suicidal beliefs' was induced. This developed category evolved from the condensing and conceptualization of two categories, namely 'Encouraging positive re-framing' and 'Gaining strength from personal beliefs'. Data provided by the participants, theoretical memos and the subsequent conceptualization of this material indicated that participants were increasingly able to assimilate information provided by the P/MH nurse and then contemplate these in relation to their own belief systems. As stated previously, suicidal people experience and interpret the world in a particular way (Shneidman 2004) and inevitably, this 'constricted' way of thinking/experiencing was different to the person's pre-suicidal patterns of thinking, feeling and behaving. The participants described how their pre-suicidal beliefs were inevitably more hopeful, indicative of the fact that they felt life was worth living and, importantly, indicative of the person's sense of feeling connected to, or part of, humanity. Accordingly, this category is concerned with the P/MH nurses' attempts to help guide the person back to these more hopeful, more connected, beliefs; supporting and encouraging the person in re-framing his/her constricted thoughts. It is concerned with helping the suicidal person re-construct a more connected and hopeful construct of the world and his/her place in it. There are at least two properties to this category. The first of these is concerned with helping suicidal people regain the support, comfort, and 'strength' of their personal belief system (whatever it may be). It is worthy of note that, on their own, such belief systems had not prevented the suicidal person from making an attempt on their life. Nevertheless, as the process of healing occurred; as the suicidal person moved more towards a 'life orientated stance', then rekindling the person's belief system was distinctly helpful for the suicidal people in this study. The second property relates to the P/MH nurse's ability to ensure the suicidal person's beliefs are kept strong through positive re-framing.

It needs to be recognized that as a community of suicidologists and mental health practitioners, we can only as yet answer a few of the most fundamental questions raised with regard to the treatment of suicide (Rudd 2000). Nevertheless, an emerging trend is distinctly noticeable among the reported empirical work that focused on short-term treatment (less than 6 months). For those studies that contain positive findings, each employed some form or version or element of cognitive behavioural therapy and each included some form of problem solving component as a core feature (Rudd 2000). Rudd (2000, p 54) continues: 'This is not particularly surprising given that CBT is perhaps the approach most amenable to a brief format'. Similarly, the work being led by Professor Paul Links, who holds the Arthur Somnerberg Chair in Suicidology at the University of Toronto, and Dr Shelley McMain from the Centre for Addictions and Mental Health, is producing similar findings. This work is producing clear positive correlations between providing care, including brief dialectic therapy as a core component, and a reduction in subsequent suicide attempts and suicidal intent. Interestingly, while not a deductive study per se, and thus not concerned with producing correlations, the findings from this current study perhaps indicate why and how these types of cognitive re-framing are of particular value for suicidal people These properties are demonstrated in the words of the study participants' words:

'The PET helped change my thoughts, helped me see that people were not against me'. (Int. S1)

'They tried to help me think differently about myself and my circumstances'. (Int. S4)

'Because my nurse stirred up different feelings, helped me change my perspective and I found this so helpful.' (Int. N2)

'I used to draw on my Christian beliefs, but even that left me when I got ill'. (Int. S1)

'I felt more powerful, felt I had got some power back at the end of the process'. (Int. N3)

'I have to focus at the moment, something tangible for the future, something to build on. That's what's driving me at the moment, giving me positive thoughts'. (Int. N1)

'I thought to myself, I'm going to fight this'. (Int. S3)

'We talked about what I thought were the positive things in my life – as well as the bad things. It was good to not just focus on the bad'. (Int. N7)

'Putting my life into a different perspective – seeing things in a different more positive way, really made a big difference'. (Int. N2)

'At first I would ridicule what I had achieved and then the PET would say, 'You should be proud of that.' (Int. S1)

'It was encouraging to know that the CAT team thought I was strong enough to get through this'. (Int. N7)

Encouraging a novel interpersonal, helping relationship

The final developed category in this sub-core variable is concerned with *encouraging a novel interpersonal, helping relationship*. Comparing new labels (new data) with existing labels and categories (existing data) enabled the preliminary category to undergo further modification and integration. As a result this developed category was induced and another was further developed, though it still retained its original name. The suicidal people in this study were clear that they gained a sense of increased hope and relief by being able to talk about their feelings, thoughts and experiences. Interestingly though, there was something qualitatively different about the relationship with the P/MH nurse, as opposed to the person's relationship with his/her family and friends, that allowed for this freedom to express, to talk frankly, and as a result, the suicidal people in this study experienced a sense of emancipation. According to the participants in this study, this freedom to reflect and talk with an experienced 'professional', in a non-judgemental atmosphere, was experienced as giving a sense of feeling very secure; the P/MH nurse had faced such situations before, knew what to do and has helped resolve similar situations previously. Thus, the relationship, though different to that in stage one, is still very important to the process and the guiding back towards humanity still occurs within the context of this relationship. The participants were also abundantly clear that, at times, they were extremely reluctant to share any of their thoughts and feelings with family or friends as they feared that this would somehow harm their significant other. Feelings are expressed sparingly within the family for fear of causing pain or risking alienation. Accordingly, the novel relationship with the P/MH nurse enabled the suicidal people to express feelings and thoughts without risking damage to their human contacts; because the P/MH nurses have been through similar before and survived, they would not be harmed (and thus neither would the person's connection with humanity).

A number of noted suicidologists, including Shneidman, Maltsberger, Maris and Leenaars for example, have noted that the relationship (and attachment) that the therapist develops is central in effective psychotherapy. This axiom is similarly applicable (and the authors of this book would argue, based on the findings of this study, that this is more applicable) to working with suicidal people. Further, we have already predicated the importance of the nurse-suicidal person relationship in phase one. However, in their excellent text, *Comprehensive Textbook of Suicidology*, Maris and colleagues (2000) draw attention to common errors of suicide interventionists:

> 'Professionalism: . . . caregivers might insulate or protect themselves from the exhausting task of empathic pairing by seeking refuge in the boundaries afforded by their role. This may overly distance and detach the caregiver and convey disinterest. Most important, it does not build upon the relationship'.
>
> Maris et al 2000, p 521

Accordingly, while an overreliance on or perhaps retreating within the boundaries of professionalism can clearly be counter-productive when working with suicidal people, it is worth noting that the suicidal people in this study drew strength from the knowledge that they were working with a mental health professional. The suicidal people placed a great deal of faith in the P/MH nurses' ability to be able to hear and deal with whatever they brought up; a dynamic that was not available to them with their family relationships. When the authors considered what were the key psychosocial processes in phase one, it became clear that part of this faith, and thus part of the sense of encountering a novel relationship, was bound up with *first* establishing the human–human contact in phase one (and thus avoiding the damaging dynamics described by Maris et al 2000). Then the suicidal people were able to gain the sense of the 'novelty' of the helping relationship and found this to be emancipatory.

Encouraging a novel interpersonal, helping relationship has at least three properties. The first is concerned with the suicidal person's need to talk through his/her problems and feelings. The second property is concerned with the ability of the P/MH nurse to receive the suicidal person's story in a manner that will not jeopardise their relationship. The third property is the P/MH nurses' ability to provide security for the suicidal person by showing experience and skill in working alongside people who feel vulnerable. These processes are described in the statements from the study participants:

Q: 'Why does listening make a difference?' A: 'It clears your mind if you can talk it over with someone else – but somebody who is not family. Family are too close'. (Int. S1)

'You can't talk to friends about some things because you want to keep them private'. (Int. N2)

'I can't talk to my wife because she doesn't really understand what I am going through'. (Int. S4)

'When you try to talk to family, or friends, there is always a kickback, so you need a professional'. (Int. N3)

'You can't explain everything to your family, you need the professional'. (Int. S3)

'I can tell the nurse things without him getting all emotional and I couldn't do that with my family and yet I needed that'. (Int. S1)

'I needed something different from 'Pull yourself together!' which is what I was getting from my family'. (Int. N2)

'You need trained people when you are in this mess. You need input from people who know what they are doing'. (Int. S3)

'I knew I had confused things in my head – and I couldn't talk to my friends about these things'. (Int. N2)

'As a result of the input from the team, they made me feel secure, and I felt as though I didn't have to rely on my family'. (Int. S3)

'It was nice just to be able to sit and chat, as I find it easier to talk to someone who doesn't know me'. (Int. N7)

THE PRELIMINARY CATEGORIES

> **Box 6.2 Guiding the Individual back to humanity (stage two): preliminary categories**
>
> M Encountering a novel interpersonal, helping relationship
> P Having personal awareness of Gestalts and moments of insight
> R Drawing strength from personal beliefs
> G Encouraging positive re-framing
> C Recognizing the limits and value of pharmacological intervention
> I Teaching and explaining

Figure 6.1 Development of the stage two categories.

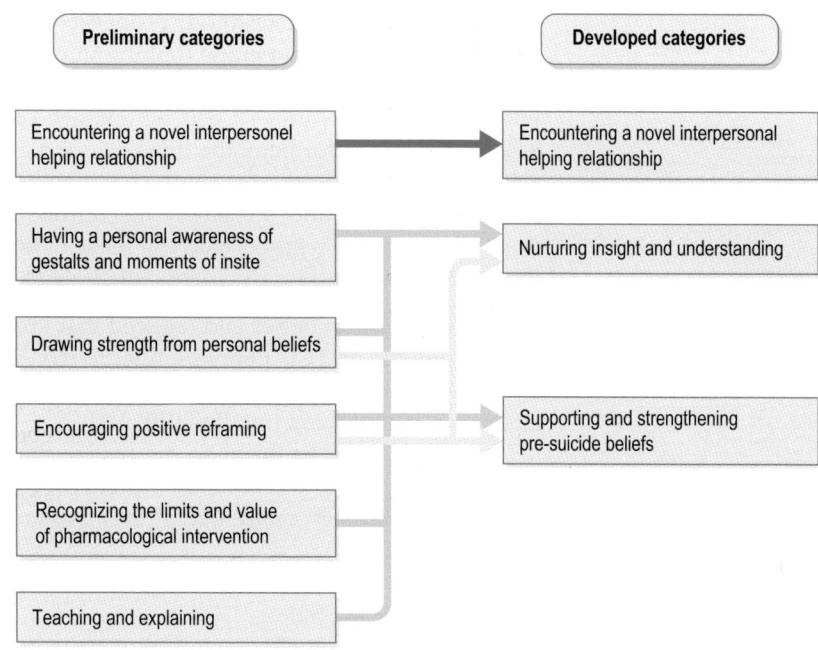

Preliminary category P: having personal awareness of Gestalts and moments of insight (re-emergence of hope)

Gestalts in this context refer to moments or 'flashes' of insight; a sudden realization of self; a hitherto unknown area or issue of self that is understood. Given that the first category in this sub-core variable '*encouraging a novel interpersonal, helping relationship*' has already been described as a developed category (see above), the next preliminary category to focus on is concerned with the increase in *Personal awareness of Gestalts and moments of insight.* In stage one, the suicidal person recognizes the reality of the suicidal act but in this category they begin to look for answers. This is perhaps evidence of the increasing contact or connection with the external world. The security offered within the novel relationship described in the previous developed category allows feelings, previously kept internalized by the suicidal person, to be discussed freely. This externalization and subsequent rationalization of these thoughts permits the suicidal person to seek understanding of their feelings. There is a growing appreciation and understanding that they do indeed need help. For some of the suicidal people in this study, this was a shocking discovery, while for others it provided a sense of relief. The suicidal people were able to externalize their actions or potential actions and to see what their suicide or suicide attempt might have been/or would be like for those close to them.

Hope begins to surface once there is recognition in the suicidal people that they needed help since this signifies a willingness to try and change their current position in life. There was an acceptance that in order to feel better the suicidal people needed to work hard, fighting their feelings, which, at times, felt like they were controlling them! The suicidal person now has more control over their destiny. The suicidal person begins to have some control over their suicidal feelings.

This category has at least four properties. The first of these is the realization within the suicidal person that the suicide attempt and/or ideation has an effect on (significant) others about them. The second property is concerned with a growing awareness and acceptance of the need for help. Having accepted the need for help, the third property refers to the suicidal person's acceptance of the 'fight' or struggle that they will need to engage in, in order to move towards, and ultimately reach, the 'life orientated' position. The final property is concerned with the sense of hope re-emerging. The following quotes from study participants illustrate these processes:

'I intended to get better and realized that I had an opportunity what with all the kindness and the people similar to me.' (Int. S3)

'Thinking about my son and what I could have done to him had a big effect on me not taking my life'. (Int. N1)

'Seeing the CAT team made me realize that somebody else recognized that I needed help and that made me feel a little better'. (Int. N7)

'I must have been really bad if they thought I needed help which was scary'. (Int. N3)

'I reached a point where I thought I have to rely on them (the PET) to help me get better'. (Int. S4)

'I acknowledged that I needed some help'. (Int. N1)

'I was ready to accept help when it was offered'. (Int. N2)

'The more I talked, the more understanding of my conflict I gained and the less likely I was to get into a downward spiral'. (Int. N3)

To conceptualize the key processes in this category, in phase one the suicidal people in this study were experiencing a sense of disconnection from the world. However, this category, *having personal awareness of Gestalts and moments of insight* suggests a re-connection with their situation and the effect of their potential actions on those about them. This is demonstrated by the range of 'guilt related' feelings illustrated within the quotes. Guilt, for some, was articulated as having a positive effect on the person at this time. It acted somewhat as an indicator to the P/MH nurse that the suicidal person was reaching out from his/her own turmoil. The P/MH nurse needed to maintain the relationship where the suicidal person is allowed to talk freely about these feelings, which, at the time could feel uncomfortable.

Preliminary category R: drawing strength from personal beliefs

This category, *Drawing strength from personal beliefs*, is concerned with the use of the suicidal person's inner beliefs and how these are accessed and used to combat his/her suicidal feelings. In essence, the suicidal person is able to harness his/her own belief system and to use this to make sense of what has happened and what they can do about it. Up until this point the suicidal person has depended on the P/MH nurse's strengths and belief in them to bolster his/her own strength, but now the suicidal person starts to re-discover his/her own abilities. There appears to be one property in this category and this is related to the comfort that the suicidal people in this study experienced as a result of re-connecting with their inner strengths. This property can be seen in the participants' comments:

'Anything that people believe in can be comforting'. (Int. S1)
'I had a lot of Christian friends come over and pray for me'. (Int. S8)
'I draw on my personal beliefs'. (Int. N1)

To conceptualize the key processes in this category, the use of personal beliefs indicates a sense of re-investing in living in that it is a re-connection with one's personal beliefs; a re-connection with the beliefs that provide meaning and strength to a person's life. Re-connecting with these beliefs can provide a sense of internal calm and possible respite from the inner turmoil that the suicidal person has experienced previously. There is also a sense that the inner strength drawn from these beliefs is dulled or even lost in the person during suicidal crisis, leaving feelings of powerlessness and hopelessness. Some participants welcomed the help from friends who share similar convictions, like the use of group prayer with Christian friends. It is interesting that closeness with a group of people with similar beliefs was important and helpful to some, while others found closeness with anyone other than the P/MH nurse difficult to deal with. Paradoxically these personal beliefs may not have value in actually discouraging the suicidal person from suicide and might strengthen the conviction in some. Take, for example, the quote below:

'Death wasn't frightening because of my beliefs'. (S1)

Personal beliefs, in this case, make suicide and death a comforting option.

Preliminary category G: encouraging positive re-framing

This next category in this sub-core variable concerns the need for the P/MH nurse to reinforce hopefulness. Listening and talking continues but now the P/MH nurse begins to highlight the positive aspects of the suicidal person and their life. This is a gentle process. The attentive P/MH nurse is vigilant to even the smallest changes in the suicidal person and his/her thoughts/feelings/behaviours. Praise and positive reinforcement are constant reminders of little achievements accomplished. There are at least two properties to this category, one of which is concerned with the P/MH nurse's ability to pick out and positively re-frame the suicidal person's strengths, even if the person can find nothing of worth in their own life. The second property is concerned with the suicidal person's ability to begin to recognize abilities in themselves and to recognize the how these strengths have been used in the past. These properties are demonstrated in the participants' own words:

'The PET team helped me focus on small goals and emphasize these as a big achievement'. (Int. S1)
'Because my nurse stirred up different feelings, helped me change my perspective and I found this so helpful'. (Int. N2)
'The PET helped change my thoughts, helped me see that people were not against me'. (Int. S1)
'Putting my life into a different perspective – seeing things in a different, more positive way, really made a difference and it was my time with my nurse and the CAT team that did that'. (Int. N2)
'They tried to help me think differently about myself and my circumstances'. (Int. S4)

It was encouraging and the reminder that I had some control, some responsibility that I could help myself'. (Int. S8)

'It was encouraging to know that the CAT team thought I was strong enough to get through this'. (Int. N7)

' . . . you have got to give yourself a pat on the back from time to time'. (Int. S1)

To conceptualize the key processes in this category, they appear to build on the process of implicit challenge from stage one. However, now the challenge begins to move from the implicit and becomes more explicit. The P/MH nurse is attempting to challenge the suicidal person's 'constriction' – the cognitive state associated with suicide. Furthermore, this process is also concerned with preparing the suicidal person for the 'meaning making' work, which occurs later in stage three. Even small changes are noticed and commented upon. By offering praise and support it is hoped that the person will gather the momentum required to move in the right direction for him/her.

Preliminary category C: recognizing the limits and value of pharmacological intervention

The next category in this sub-core variable is concerned with *recognizing the limitations of pharmacological intervention*. This category illustrates the value and the problems associated with the medication used to help people who are feeling suicidal. Medication did have a place for some of the suicidal people in this study, it helped them 'feel fine', 'be more in control', 'lift mood' and 'aid sleep'. However and importantly, focusing on medication and pharmacological intervention was just what some participants did not want. Such an emphasis had a sense of losing the person in the search for the 'brain'. Accordingly, in some cases, this gave the suicidal people in this study a further sense of being disconnected from humanity. For others, medication was fraught with side effects, which served only to increase, not decrease their psychache and anxiety. Having gained a level of personal control in their life, the suicidal people were disturbed by medication causing an altered level of mental functioning. This is especially true if medication meant that the suicidal people were unable to resume their normal activities. The suicidal people in this study made it clear that medication is only one part of the suicidal person's care and it is not always suitable for everyone. Medication needs to be supplemented with time, talk and therapy. Consequently, the process in this category was recognizing that medication is only one treatment available, and, for the participants in this study, did not appear to be enough on its own.

There are at least three properties to this category. The first property is concerned with the recognition that the 'answer' or 'solution' to the suicidal crisis did not reside in a 'pill'. There was no 'magic bullet' drug that the suicidal people could take that would make their situation change. The participants in this study wanted more than simply being offered another drug or having their drugs changed. This inappropriate emphasis, at times, gave the participants a further sense of being disconnected from humanity. The second property is concerned with recognizing that even the periods of relief that were experienced for some, were offset in the longer term, as a result of the severe and debilitating side-effects experienced. The third property is concerned with recognizing that, in some cases, certain medications provided periods of relief. This was most often relief from stress, sleeplessness and the sense of lack of control. These processes were described and captured by the participants in the following ways:

'I would not have got better if all I had received was more tablets'. (Int. S3)

'I saw the doctor and he put me on an anti-depressant, but I said to him that I really needed some counselling'. (Int. N2)

'My GP was going to give me more tablets, but my daughter insisted that this wasn't enough for me, that I needed more help and she was right'. (Int. S3)

'Them three weeks, as I waited for the anti-depressants to kick in, were a long three weeks'. (Int. S1)

'I had been prescribed Diazepam to help me sleep, but these were not working and I ended up taking lots of them at once'. (Int. S3)

'The doctors prescribed me some Peroxatine, and I started to take those, but the side effects kick in bad enough for me not to be able to go to work'. (Int. N5)

'I was given tablets to help me sleep. They were all right at first but they gave me side effects'. (Int. S2)

'The drugs just seemed to make me more anxious and upset than ever. I didn't feel they were helping me in the least'. (Int. S8)

'I don't want knocking out from morning to night'. (Int. S1)

'I felt in more control after my medication was changed'. (Int. S4)

'Obviously, the tablets started to kick in and I did feel fine'. (Int. N8)

'Getting the right medication was important to me'. (Int. S4)

'The tablets did me some good in that they calmed me down'. (Int. S1)

To conceptualize the key processes in this category, as stated above, focusing on medication and pharmacological intervention was just what some suicidal people did not want. Such an emphasis had a sense of losing the person in the search for the 'brain'. Accordingly, in some cases, this gave the participants a further sense of being disconnected from humanity. Consequently, what is clearly happening in this category is recognizing (and acting accordingly) that the P/MH nurse needs to focus on the person – not the medication. Further recognizing that side effects can also serve to reinforce the sense of being disconnected once more prompts the P/MH nurse to focus on the person. Essentially this category is about conceptualizing the 'place' that medication has in the care of the suicidal person. It is a limited place, an adjunct place, a short-term crisis role. Not the principal and pivotal role that medication is often posited as having.

Preliminary category I: teaching and explaining

The final preliminary category in this sub-core variable is concerned with the P/MH nurse *teaching and explaining* what has happened to the suicidal people, what will happen and what tools can be used to lessen problems. Teaching and explaining occurs throughout stage two. The suicidal people in this study wanted to know what was going to happen to them, and they wanted these explanations. In some cases, as they had never experienced a service like this before, they were unsure what to expect. There is a well established body of evidence that indicates how informing people can reduce anxiety (and stress). Thus, it is not surprising that being more informed, having a sense of what was to come and the concomitant reduction in stress, helped to move the suicidal people in this study back towards a 'life orientated' position. In addition to providing answers to questions and explaining what was ahead, the P/MH nurses also engaged in specific 'teaching strategies' to equip the suicidal people with more 'tools' to help combat their suicidal thoughts/feelings. Again, many of these were 'stress reduction' techniques and/or 'anxiety' management techniques. It is noteworthy that attempts to teach or provide the suicidal people with such 'tools' did not happen in phase one. The suicidal people in this study were not at a place psychologically, during stage one, where they would be able to assimilate the 'teaching'; to attempt to teach someone when they are disconnected from humanity would be the height of folly. However, once the person has re-established the first tenuous connections with humanity, then they become more amenable to receiving appropriate, helpful information and tools.

There are at least three properties to this category *Teaching and explaining*. The first property describes the participants' requests for information. The second is concerned with the way the suicidal people chose to use the information that they were given. The final property is about the ability of the P/MH nurses to match need with the right sort of information at the right time. These processes were described and captured by the participants in the following ways:

'The PET gave me a list of what we were going to do'. (Int. S1)

'They explained things to me'. (Int. S4)

'They gave me handouts and information on the signs and symptoms of anxiety'. (Int. S3)

'Any and everything they were going to do with me they explained'. (Int. S4)

'They taught me how to relax, how to meditate and showed me what anxiety was'. (Int. S3)

'They (PET) taught me how to deal with my anxiety attacks and shortness of breath'. (Int. S1)

'When I first went to the services what I wanted from people were some tools. I didn't want a magic wand. If there is fine, fine, wave it by all means but given that there isn't one a magic wand, then give me tools, or suggest some tools, show me some tools. Those were the things I wasn't being given before.' (Int. N5)

To conceptualize the key processes in this category, there is a clear sense that this category is concerned with providing the person with some of the 'tools' that can help the suicidal person re-connect with humanity. This category indicates that the process is beginning to move away from connecting exclusively with the P/MH nurse (as this has already occurred) and is now shifting the emphasis to connecting with other people as well. It is concerned with helping the suicidal person feel less powerless; less at the mercy of previous constricting thoughts/feelings. In feeling more empowered, in feeling more capable to be around others, the person can connect more easily. This category is also about helping the suicidal people to learn that what they are experiencing is very common. Thus, having these experiences does not make the suicidal person more 'odd' and thus more disconnected from the rest of humanity. On the contrary, it teaches the suicidal person that what they are experiencing is synonymous with being human.

Chapter 7

Learning to Live – Stage Three

'Every minute I was there, they were bringing me back to the land of the living – not the land of the dead.'
Interview S3

CHAPTER CONTENTS

INTRODUCTION

In this chapter we provide a detailed further description and additional explanation of the specific qualities, interventions and activities that the P/MH nurse can use in order to provide meaningful care for the suicidal person in this stage of the process. As stated in the previous chapter, processes occur over time, thus this chapter is concerned with the third of such stages: the third and final sub-core variable of our findings and subsequent theory. This stage was termed '*Learning to live*' and it captures the third phase of providing meaningful, therapeutic, transformative care for the suicidal individual.

We begin this chapter by providing an overview of the third stage and this is further illustrated by drawing heavily on direct quotes provided by the participants. We follow this with a more detailed explanation of the two key psychosocial processes (which represent the developed or de-limited theoretical categories) subsumed within this stage. These are termed: '*Accommodating an existential crisis, past, present and future*' and '*Going on in the context set by the existential relationship with suicide*'. Each of these is also explained and evidenced by drawing on direct quotes from the participants. In turn, these categories were developed and modified from four preliminary categories, therefore, we also describe, explain and substantiate each of these, and once again, support them with direct quotes. In order to help understand the construction and development of the findings, the developed and preliminary categories are listed in Boxes 7.1 and 7.2, respectively, and depicted in Figure 7.1. Accordingly, after reading this chapter, the practitioner should be more aware the range of specific qualities, interventions and activities that the P/MH nurses used in phase three, and the suicidal people found to be of immense value and help. Further, the reader should be able to understand both the empirical background and theoretical development of these ways of working with suicidal people. As a result the findings should have more credibility, more spontaneous validity and more, to paraphrase Glaser (1978), fit and grab.

OVERVIEW

This sub-core variable '*Learning to live*' is the third stage of 'Re-connecting the person with humanity', or to rephrase, the third stage providing meaningful, therapeutic, transformative care for the suicidal people in this study is actualized through a combination of two developed categories. The sub-core variable 'Learning to live' is concerned with how suicidal people begin to pick up the threads of their life, and how the professional (P/MH nurse) response continues to have a place; although this is somewhat different to that of earlier stages. In stage two., the P/MH nurse is walking with the suicidal person, setting the scene for re-connecting with humanity through positive re-framing, teaching and explaining, capitalizing on personal awareness moments etc. In stage three the P/MH nurse adopts the role of 'wise consultant'. However, the P/MH nurse must also be prepared to let the suicidal people engage with their own 'sense making' in relation to their suicidality, as this remains an existential crisis. The importance of sense making in relation to suicide has been recognized by Albert Camus (1945):

> *'There is but one serious philosophical problem, and that is suicide. Judging whether life is or is not worth living amounts to answering the fundamental question of philosophy.'*

The suicidal people in this study were undertaking momentous work and so it is not surprising that, at times, they become overwhelmed and need to turn to the P/MH nurse for help. At this stage, however, the P/MH nurse is a source of expert advice and not simply a co-presence. Early challenges to negative perceptions would be too difficult to accommodate in the context of the loss of humanity and general rawness the person is experiencing. But, the experience of P/MH nurse 'co-presencing' and the reflecting of humanity prepared the ground for more structured and directive work. The P/MH nurses recognized that they cannot impose their meaning on the suicidality for it is deeply personal and individual. The P/MH nurse's counsel was offered, but would not always be accepted as the suicidal people fitted together a story that accounts for the way in which their suicidality came into their life, its place in the here and now and its trajectory into the future – hard and demanding and long-term work.

Understanding the suicidality helped the suicidal people in this study feel more in control. Personal understanding allows the suicidal people to re-engage more fully with people other than the professionals. The suicidal people in this study were often reluctant to discuss their thought/actions with significant others; there are varied reasons for this. Sometimes, it is because their suicidality seems like a 'private function'. Alternatively, there was evidence of a belief that other people could not appreciate or understand something the suicidal people themselves could not account for. In stage three the suicidal people in this study revisited their decision to engage with suicidality. The re-appraisal took place in relation to whether life was, is and will be worth living, and involved re-visiting many factors, for example, their degree of connectedness with others. A re-working of previous assessments occurred, for example, in relation to whether or not the suicidal person would be missed, and the effect the suicide would have had and would have if executed in the here and now. At this stage, there is a focus on how a worthwhile life can be re-established.

An important process in this phase, and one concerned with re-establishing the suicidal person's re-investment in life, is 'doing' as well as 'talking'. Sometimes, the P/MH nurses would encourage the suicidal people to engage in practical activity. Small successes can also help the suicidal people to gain power over their suicidality, because even very basic everyday activities, at times, seemed impossible to achieve. The 'doing' helps the suicidal people to feel more hopeful. It offers a counterpoint to the difficult, thoughtful work that the suicidal people were undertaking in relation to their suicide attempt. While it is tempting for all concerned to think of the suicidality as an entirely negative phenomenon, for some of the suicidal people in this study it was more complex than that. Some of the participants in this study referred to how their suicidality could have a place as 'friend' and 'foe' for them. While the P/MH nurse may hope for the suicidality to depart from the suicidal person's life, there are, at times and for some of the suicidal people in this study, good reasons for them to maintain a relationship with it. However, the suicidal people in this study were clear that their relationship with their suicidality needed to be one in which they had a sense of power and control over the suicidality, if it was to have a positive as well as potentially negative function for them. The basic psychosocial processes of the sub-core variable were expressed by participants in the following ways:

'It feels fabulous to be doing these normal, everyday things again, because I had stopped doing them.' (Int. S3)

'I couldn't handle more challenge early on. It would have been too much. I needed people to be nice to me. I needed everything from the cotton wool world.' (Int. N3)

'So there is a time for challenging constructions of hopelessness and negative, limiting constructs and there is a time for leaving well alone and providing another way of help.' (Int. N1)

'Talking to my CPN helped me gain a different perspective on the significant events. Instead of seeing the bad and feeling disconnected from my family, I was able to see the good, feel compassion, and feel more connected with her (daughter).' (Int. S3)

'He suggested things like imagining the top of my head was open and I could put my hand in and pull out my problems and pull out the tension and put it on the table – just things like that. But there was also lots of praise, 'well done, you went in and you tried it, well done'. Lots of praise. 'You are top man'. A lot of what the nurses are doing you can see why they are doing it. It is overt help, but it doesn't feel false. It is genuine. It is trained. It is their job, they are saying things they are trained to say, but, what the hell, it feels fine.' (Int. N5)

'(The feeling less suicidal) is not clear-cut or the kind of process that makes you suddenly think 'I want to live'. It is extremely difficult to work out what they did or said. But they did stop me wanting to die, stopped me doing anything about it'. (Int. N3)

'He (nurse) encouraged me, said positive things to me; encouraged me to attend to the small things, like washing, shaving.' (Int. S4)

'It was four or five weeks when I came back a bit.' (Int. N3)

'Six weeks ago, I could not have gone out with the kids – but now it has shifted.' (Int. N3)

'My thread was not wanting my kids to end up traumatised by my suicide.' (Int. N3)

'It was like feeling a bit more in line with society again. I felt a bit more in line with the usual. This made me feel a bit better.' (Int. S8)

'(I think of my possible suicide as) An enemy, because you are doing something to yourself which is going to cause so much heartache to other people (my son and parents). But I couldn't live with the way my life was going at the time; I couldn't handle it any more. . . That side was a good side of it, if there was one, because it was a way out of my problems.' (Int. N7)

'The feeling (suicidal feelings) never goes away – it is there at the back of my head all the time.' (Int. N8)

THE DEVELOPED CATEGORIES

> **Box 7.1 Learning to live (stage three): developed categories**
>
> ■ Accomodating an existential crisis, past, present and future
> ■ Going on in the context set by the existential relationship with suicide

Accommodating an existential crisis, past, present and future

Comparing new labels and existing labels and categories enabled the preliminary categories to undergo further modification and integration. As a result two new developed categories were induced. The first of these is accommodating an existential crisis, past, present and future. Certain preliminary categories (namely: *Experiencing a sense of post-suicidal support, and Embracing the hard work of re-investing in living*) indicated that each appeared to contain a similar process or processes to one another, and these common processes thus indicated the properties of the category. The similar indicated that, rather than dismissing the suicidality, it had to be made sense of in a complex way. Further, that this 'sense making' would be achieved through an array of interpersonal processes, including supportive involvement from professionals (mainly P/MH nurses in this study), family and fellow travellers on the suicidality path. These processes indicated at least two properties of the category. First, there is a property concerned with dealing with existential angst. Existential crises concern facing up to the realities of living and dying in the context of the inevitability of dying. The suicidal person has somehow 'short-circuited' the normal trajectory and come to face his/her own mortality in a dramatic way. Nothing can ever be the same again, and it is naïve of P/MH nurses to look for the return to the person's pre-suicide state. Consequently, the process of sense making is still relevant and less academic than for many other people. Important 'self-searching' questions that the suicidal people in this study asked themselves (directly or indirectly) included,

'How could I have reached such a place?'
'Why did I feel so far away from those I love?'
'How do I explain to them what I tried to do?'
'How do I going on living the rest of my life knowing I tried to commit suicide?'
'How can I use this experience so that I don't end up here again?'
'Maybe some good will come of this? Maybe there will come a time when I won't have to do this again?'

Thus, if suicidal people can arrive at a satisfactory account; if they can consider these questions (and their own individual set of sense making questions), then it is possible to have some power over their relationship with suicidality. In some ways, for the suicidal people in this study, their relationship with death was, in a somewhat counter-intuitive or paradoxical way, more empowering than that afforded to many other people, provided that it can be kept in its place. Their attempt at suicide became a reminder of what could happen when life became difficult. Their attempt served as an *aide mémoire* of a course of action that had been 'tried out' and found to be lacking; as a result it helped the suicidal people opt for 'life choices' rather than 'death choices'; it helped them engage in more rational and informed choices.

The second property is concerned with how the individual resolution of the existential crisis is moderated by significant others, both professional and family. There is a rhythm of support established between suicidal person, family and P/MH nurses. Of course, dealing with an existential crisis is hard, tiring and lengthy work. It necessarily has to be undertaken by the suicidal person in a 'private space'. However, the P/MH nurse's co-presence and experience serves to keep the suicidal person anchored, even if this presence is virtual rather than physical, and the suicidal people in this study used this 'sense of being anchored' as the platform from which to begin their re-connection with humanity. Without protracted contact and support from the P/MH nurse, the suicidal people were in danger of feeling that nothing is real except their own thought processes; leading to what Sartre would describe as 'Nothingness', the antithesis of 'Being'. As the suicidal people acknowledged the effects of their suicidal act on others, they were starting (already) to move forward from their existential crisis, in that there was an acknowledgement of their attachment to the world; a growing acknowledgment that they were (and are) connected to others in the world. The drastic and dramatic effects of the suicidality in the past, present and future thus can act as a deterrent against future suicide attempts. Being at least partially re-connected with humanity brings with it a peril. The P/MH nurse's withdrawal can be experienced as a rejection. Accordingly, and as with many other therapeutic relationships (Peplau 1988) the end of the relationship may need to be gradual, delayed, protracted and managed, so that the suicidal people feel that they are letting go; so that they don't feel that the P/MH nurse has simply lost interest in them or is ignorant of the ongoing management of life post-suicidality. In this context, it is not surprising that the suicidal people in this study were open to contact with others who have or are addressing the place of suicidality in their lives. These properties are expressed and captured in the participants' own words:

'(The feeling less suicidal) is not clear-cut, or the kind of process that makes you suddenly think, 'I want to live'. It is extremely difficult to work out what they did or said. But they did stop me wanting to die, stopped me doing anything about it.' (Int. N3)

'Every minute I was there, they were bringing me back to the land of the living – not the land of the dead.' (Int. S3)

'Talking to my C.P.N. helped me gain a different perspective on the significant events.' (Int. N2)

'The feeling (suicidal feelings) never go away – it is there, at the back of my head all the time.' (Int. N8)

'If I get suicidal thoughts now I try to push them out. I also think about the repercussions on those I leave behind and this helps stop me do it.' (Int. N7)

'I wanted the contact with my nurse to go on longer.' (Int. S8)

'I had to re-establish a connection with my daughter and her family after talking with my nurse.' (Int. N2)

'If I get suicidal thoughts now I try to push them out. I also think about the repercussions on those I leave behind and this helps stop me do it.' (Int. N7)

'It is hard to explain to your family why you have done what you have; they don't understand.' (Int. N4)

'Instead of seeing the bad and feeling disconnected from my family, I was able to see the good, feel compassion and feel more connected with her (daughter).' (Int. N2)

'By the time those two women (CPNs) left, I was looking less miserable, less desperate.' (Int. N3)

'The only support I was getting was from my nurse and the CAT team and I was scared about not seeing him any longer; no longer having this support.' (Int. S2)

'It was easy to give up, so re-connecting was scary.' (Int. N3)

'I felt there was a thread keeping me on this planet.' (Int. N3)

'I now view or describe my suicidal feelings as an option that I have closed the lid on, something like closing a box. . .I keep this box in the back of my head, right at the back in the attic.' (Int. N8)

'It is the fact that I am not the only one. I am not on my own – that there are other people like me.' (Int. N4)

'It is scary picking up the pieces, but I needed to. I wanted to make sure I wouldn't reach this place again.' (Int. S3)

'You have to deal with what had gone on.' (Int. S8)

Going on in the context set by the existential relationship with suicidality

Through a process of modification and integration of preliminary categories a developed category was induced titled 'Going on in the context set by the existential relationship with suicidality'. Specific categories that contributed were: Re-engaging in the ordinariness of life; Re-emerging hope. Each of these preliminary categories appeared to contain similar processes to the other, and these indicated the properties of the new category. First, there is a property concerned with how, for the suicidal people in this study, life gradually became more balanced between extremes. Possible extremes were: life and death, physical and emotional care, co-presence and direction, professional support and family support, hopelessness and hopefulness. For the suicidal people in this study who were attempting to make sense of their suicidality, it was important to have the hard emotional work balanced by the practical. To a great extent, practically living life seemed to be helpful in accommodating the existential crisis; this practical, 'day to day' living also provided a context for the 'sense making' work. This 'day to day' life was, after all, the life the suicidal person would need to go on living. This was the context into which the experience of suicide would now have to be woven. The engagement in the practical re-invests life with a sense of normality and this helps the suicidal person to feel re-connected with humanity. In tandem, the P/MH nurse needed to offer different types of support. In relation to emotional support, she/he needed to offer both co-presence and some more challenging input. In relation to practical support, the P/MH nurse is an 'encourager', helping the suicidal person to do very basic things and also to engage in displacement activity, e.g., swimming. The combination of extremes helps the suicidal people 'go on' with their life.

Similarly, the role of significant others becomes balanced. In the period before the suicide attempt and aftermath, the suicidal people in this study had been reluctant to speak with their family members. This seems to be so that the family's feelings are spared and because there is a sense of disbelief that anyone can understand what the suicidal people cannot understand themselves. To some extent, this accounts for why the P/MH nurses, with their special experience of people in suicidality, were a more welcome co-respondent. However, as the suicidal people undertook the work associated with their existential crisis, their own understanding of past, present and future life appeared to increase. With the increased understanding, the suicidal people gained more capacity to hold the lack of understanding of others. Being able to be absorb the needs of significant others allows more sense of connection and the opportunity to connect with humanity.

In tandem to the increased everyday activity, and the re-connection with family, the suicidal people in this study experienced a resurgence of hope. In particular, as the suicidal people began to resolve some of their existential crisis there was an increased feeling of hopefulness. However, hope was related also to the more mundane aspects of living. As the suicidality had interrupted the flow of everyday living so dramatically, the re-institution of even very basic life skills becomes a barometer of hope. Thus, the role of the P/MH nurse in helping suicidal people re-establish 'the basics', and recognize the small changes that are occurring should not be underestimated. Competence in the 'here and now' also helps with a re-evaluation of the past and present. Hope develops in an upward spiral, that itself helps to control the suicidality. These properties are expressed and captured in the participants' own words:

'I could do with someone to help me get going, like going swimming, help me with my weights, do stuff together, maybe even help me get a job.' (Int. S2)

'Just progress in the small things, like putting some smart clothes on, boosted me up.' (Int. S4)

'The good ones (nurses) will take you out, take you for a drive, go for a coffee.' (Int. S2)

'I was scared when I cooked again for the first time, so I cried. I was pleased but I was still scared.' (Int. S1)

'I started to take some positive steps, tried to reconnect, like sending a letter.' (Int. N2)

'My connection was, and is, the kids.' (Int. N3)

'Now, as I start to feel better, I would like to see what the next 50 years hold.' (Int. N3)

'I am more hopeful that I have a future and maybe that everything is not as bad as I think it is.' (Int. N7)

Figure 7.1 Development of the stage three categories.

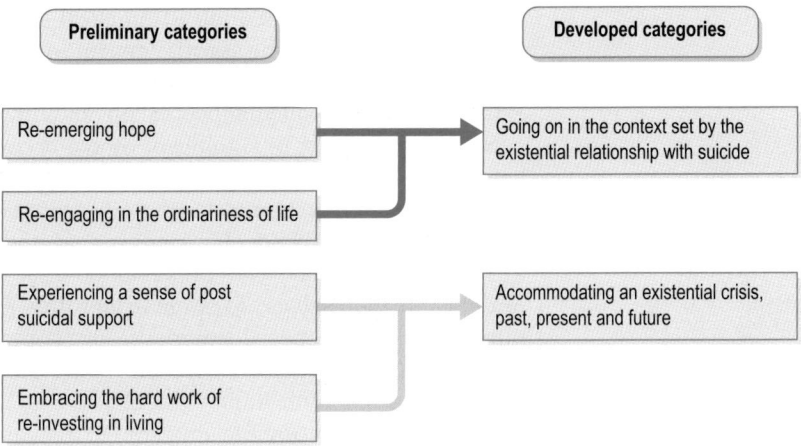

THE PRELIMINARY CATEGORIES

Box 7.2 Learning to live (stage three): preliminary categories

N Re-emerging hope
A Re-engaging in the ordinariness of life
K Experiencing a sense of post-suicidal support
S Embracing the hard work of re-investing in living

Preliminary category N: re-emerging hope

The first preliminary category in the sub-core variable 'Learning to live' is concerned with *Re-emerging hope*. In essence, this category illustrates and explains the process whereby the suicidal people began to feel more hopeful; even acknowledging that they were becoming more hopeful. It is also concerned with how this increased sense of hopefulness helped the suicidal people begin to try to establish some control over the role of suicidality in their life. In the previous stages, the suicidal people had relied on the P/MH nurse to help control suicidality, although the seeds of hope have been sown during stage two. During stage three, however, they are taking up responsibility and developing hope. Yet, the suicidal people in this study described how hope fluctuates rather than growing incrementally in a linear way. Thus, it is not surprising that the suicidal people in this study talked of needing continued P/MH nursing assistance to give them a boost when the going gets tough.

The suicidal people in this study described how in the past suicidality has loomed large; not surprisingly they wanted to gain some power over it. Doing and recognizing the change in everyday activity in the 'here and now' (see below) helped the suicidal people to become more in control and more hopeful. The strength to carry on and re-engage with life activities can be derived from future or present oriented factors. The suicidal people in this study described the usefulness of having goals to aim for. Others described an inner life force that they drew upon.

This category contains at least two properties. The first property is concerned with the suicidal people becoming more hopeful and thus gaining more power and control over their suicidality; it describes the change in belief regarding the inevitability of the suicide and feelings of distress. The second property is concerned with past, present and future orienting. Positive events in the 'here and now' and possible future aid a re-appraisal of the role of suicidality in the suicidal person's life. The following quotes illustrate the properties:

'Regaining my previous activities and abilities gave me hope.' (Int. S3)

'(After talking with my nurse) I felt that my positive feelings had been stirred up.' (Int. N2)

'I felt more powerful, felt I had got some power back at the end of the process.' (Int. N3)

'I started to believe I would get better. I became more hopeful. I got hope and I felt positive.' (Int. S8)

'I started to think, 'Maybe there will come a time when I won't have to do this again.' (Int. N8)

'Some days I have more hope now.' (Int. N8)

'The exams gave me some goal – something to aim for, some focus.' (Int. S8)

'I have a focus at the moment, something tangible for the future, something to build on, that's what's driving me on at the moment, giving me positive thoughts.' (Int. N1)

'I draw on my inner strength.' (Int. N1)

To conceptualize the key processes in this category, they are those of describing the way in which hope re-emerges in conjunction with the suicidal person's growing sense of power over the suicidality. The suicidality has interrupted the suicidal person's life in every sense. Even ordinary, taken-for-granted activities have been a challenge. Power over the suicidality can be sourced from internal or external sources. The P/MH nurse has a function of stirring up positive feelings, drawing on present and future possibilities. The P/MH nurse can do so from a connection with the suicidal person, that has been established in stages one and two that allows the person to hear the P/MH nurse's wisdom. One means of doing this is to identify the small changes that are already occurring for the suicidal person, in relation to his/her capacity to re-engage with the tasks of every day life. Success in small tasks allows hope for the future, and this is manifested as hope in the present. As hope re-emerges, there is a sense in which the suicidality can be kept in its place and that a suicide attempt will not recur.

Preliminary category A: re-engaging in the ordinariness of life

The next preliminary category in this sub-core variable, 'Learning to live', is concerned with *Re-engaging in the ordinariness of life*. In essence, this category illustrates and explains the processes where the P/MH nurse helps the suicidal person to function at a basic level in ensuring that simple needs are fulfilled. Routines of everyday living are a necessity. *Doing* normal things can make the suicidal person *feel* more normal and so more connected to humanity. Physical activity is described as a welcome distraction from the suicidality. Doing small everyday things counterbalances the search for meaning that the suicidal person is undertaking in relation to the suicide attempt. For some of the suicidal people in this study the emotional work is balanced by physical 'work'.

In stage three, the suicidal people in this study continue to be aware of the need of co-presence when the humanity of the P/MH nurse is still sustaining, and the more structured involvement that the P/MH nurse offers in tandem. However, participants in this study described beginning to link more with other people. Family, friends and fellow travellers on the path to understanding suicidality are all possible connections. Being a 'helper' also serves as a connector. The category contains at least two properties. The first property is concerned with the process of being grounded to humanity by engaging in everyday activities; beginning to feel normal again and balancing the hard emotional work post suicide attempt. The second property is concerned with re-establishing a connection with significant others; through this, the suicidal people gained a sense of their worth as a person. The following quotes illustrate these properties:

'They would bring me things to give me options for things to do (practically) in the future.' (Int. S3)

'I wanted and needed to get back to basics, something to eat, something to drink, getting back to the basic process of what, to me, being a man is about.' (Int. N1)

'I would have liked to have done more things with people, you know, go out more, go places.' (Int. S2)

'I needed people with me – I needed both practical and emotional support for day to day functioning.' (Int. N3)

'Now (post professional input) I do things that my mind can deal with, simple things. But it keeps me busy instead of allowing my mind to go blank.' (Int. S3)

'I could look forward to him coming – having a laugh and a joke, taking me out, making sure I didn't feel low, because if I did he would pick me up again.' (Int. N8)

'I had to re-establish a connection with my daughter and her family after talking with my nurse.' (Int. N2)

'Talking to someone else who had gone through the same problem helps you to feel that you are not alone.' (Int. S3)

'Extra support would have helped, even from a volunteer.' (Int. N2)

'It made me feel a lot better to go to meeting where I could recognize a lot of other people's problems as being similar to my own.' (Int. N4)

'I think that having gone through this myself, I would be able to help others in the same situation.' (Int. S8)

'I have joined various volunteer groups that help other people.' (Int. S3)

'My CPN would encourage me to do active things and help me do this. This helped.' (Int. S4)

To conceptualize the key processes in this category, they are those of creating a context in which basic physical and social needs can be met which engender a sense of normality and so a sense of re-connecting with humanity. The P/MH nurse is still fulfilling a function, and must retain a presence although doing so differently. If the social network is poor, the P/MH nurse may need to be able to 'toggle' between being a friend for the suicidal person (engaging in everyday activities) and offering a more professional 'face'. The P/MH nurse needs to take a complementary role of 'balanced supporting'. As the suicidal people strive to make sense of their suicidality, they need a complementary practical focus otherwise the emotional work would be too intense. Working solely on the meaning of the suicidality can lead the suicidal person to feel confused or without ideas – blank. The P/MH nurse is an 'encourager' offering ideas and options to energize the suicidal person. In the early stages after the experience of suicidality, the suicidal people in this study felt most at home in the company of strangers; albeit ones who can co-presence. This spares the feelings of the suicidal person's loved ones, who may be struggling to understand the person's motives and emotions, while dealing with their own reaction to the suicide attempt. To re-connect, involves a widening of the previously more exclusive helping relationship(s) with the professional system and more opportunity to confirm her/his own humanity.

Preliminary category K: experiencing a sense of post suicidal support

The next preliminary category in the sub-core variable, 'Learning to live', is concerned with *Experiencing a sense of post-suicidal support*. The suicidal people in this study described the need for complimentary external support as they were working on their relationship with suicidality and 'meaning making'. Often, they reported wanting support to be regular and intensive, as in stage one. The suicidal people in this study valued the option of having a responsive P/MH nurse as 'back up'. Sometimes, simply knowing that the P/MH nurse is a telephone call away was sufficient. However, when the relationship with suicidality becomes intrusive, the P/MH nurse's willingness to act more directly to help the suicidal person to exert some control over it was welcome. This allows the suicidal person to feel safer and less alone.

At this stage, the suicidal people in the study described their family offering support also. Despite this, the participants distinguished the need for ongoing involvement from their P/MH nurse and stated their preference for a slow 'weaning off' from their P/MH nursing network. This category contains at least one property. It is concerned with the variety of the helping relationship; whether this is professional or family and how this organized; the frequency and length of involvement. The following quotes illustrate these properties:

'(When the support was absent) I felt left alone, like I had to get through it on my own.' (Int. S2)
'It was nice to see someone who understands and it was nice to see someone regularly.' (Int. S8)
'I felt safer with the CAT team.' (Int. N3)
'Anytime I needed support they came out to me.' (Int. S4)
'I needed someone to talk to and I felt I could call on them at any time.' (Int. S2)
'(When the support was absent) I felt left alone like I had to get through it on my own.' (Int. S2)

'There was always someone at hand, just a phone call away.' (Int. N1)

'I was told that if I needed help, I should call his secretary and she would put me through, so that made me feel safe. . .I felt like I had a safety net there.' (Int. N2)

'But just knowing they were there – that was the difference.' (Int. N8)

'It's knowing that someone is there.' (Int. S2)

'They had to discharge me and they asked me if I was all right with that. I said, 'Yes, I have the (CAT team) phone number.' (Int. N8)

'My family make sure that I'm alright.' (Int. S2)

'My mother was coming to us (and support) me as well.' (Int. S7)

'My family came and gave me support, helped out in the house and talked with me.' (Int. N3)

'I felt really scared about being left on my own, because I didn't have any support.' (Int. N2)

'There was a seamless transition from nurse to nurse after the attempt, a gradual withdrawal and a change in the nature of support.' (Int. N3)

'At first I felt a little distraught at the sudden ending . . . . . . I wanted more time and longer time with the PET.' (Int. S1)

'I wanted the PET to stay a bit longer the second time in case something happened.' (Int. S4)

'I could have done with someone coming to see me for longer.' (Int. S2)

'The contact with the PET team should be longer and not cut off so quickly.' (Int. S1)

To conceptualize the key processes in this category, they are those of establishing a rhythm between the suicidal person, the P/MH nurse and family in relation to support. The suicidal people have to have space to do their suicidality work in private. It cannot be accomplished by the P/MH nurse on their behalf. However, it was very clear that the P/MH nurse still had a major function to fulfil. Co-presence is carried through from stage one, but now the presence may not necessarily need to be physical. The suicidal people feel the security at a distance, even when the P/MH nurse is absent, although only a phone call away. This re-connection with humanity is part of an upward spiral, the opposite of the downturn that the suicidality, secrecy and disconnection from family members represented. Perhaps the suicidal person is now more able to make sense of the suicidality and so can be with people who may still be struggling to understand. The relationship with suicidality is ongoing. Consequently, ending must be gradual, rather than the suicidal person feeling that the P/MH nurse has lost interest or does not understand the complexities of managing life post-suicidality.

Preliminary category S: embracing the hard work of re–investing in living

The next preliminary category in the (sub) core variable, 'Learning to live', is concerned with *Embracing the hard work of re-investing in living*. The suicidal people in this study made reference to having to accept that the suicide would not disappear overnight. They saw it very much as a process rather than there being a point of reference. Indeed, the suicidal people in this study seemed to accept that the suicidality would remain with them even if it was in a different form or contained in some way. The mechanisms of containment were varied, as disclosed by the participants. For example, the suicidality can be 'boxed up'. The suicidal people in this study described the complex ways in which they related to suicidality for example as a 'way out' (a friend) or a 'guilt giver' (a foe). They spoke of the repercussions of a successful and unsuccessful attempt. If successful, there are people left behind (although there was acknowledgement that being in suicidality made the suicidal people think that those left would be better off without them). If it is not successful the suicidal people have to face the fact that they would have been missed by their significant others. In all cases, the suicidal people talked about the hard work of re-investing. It is an uphill struggle, and suicidal people need sustaining on the journey.

This category contains at least two properties. The first property is concerned with constructing the meaning(s) of suicidality in the past, present and future. The second property is concerned with the hard work that discerning meaning involves and how the work is sustained. The following quotes illustrate these properties:

'(The feeling less suicidal) is not clear-cut, or the kind of process that makes you suddenly think, 'I want to live'. It is extremely difficult to work out what they did or said. But they did stop me wanting to die, stopped me doing anything about it.' (Int. N3)

'The feeling (suicidal feelings) never go away – it is there, at the back of my head all the time.' (Int. N8)

'If I get suicidal thoughts now I try to push them out. I also think about the repercussions on those I leave behind and this helps stop me do it.' (Int. N7)

'My thread was not wanting my kids to end up traumatised by my suicide.' (Int. N3)

'Sometimes my suicidality is a 'friend', sometimes it is an 'enemy' but it is an option; it will always be an option . . . . . . my relationship with my suicide is now like a person that is always with me.' (Int. N8)

'So while it (suicide option) stays with me, I can manage it in different ways.' (Int. N8)

'I just want to shut the lid on it (suicidality) and keep it shut.' (Int. N8)

'I sometimes look at the (security) plan I had made and look at my pills and this stops me doing it as it makes me think the consequences out.' (Int. S1)

'When I am asked how I know I am not going to do it now, I say, 'I have to think of those other three'.' (Int. N8)

'I sometimes think that because I didn't do it (commit suicide) this might help me not do it again. So, it has helped me that way.' (Int. N8)

'The recovery is the hard part.' (Int. N3)

'It was easy to give up, so re-connecting was scary.' (Int. N3)

'I acknowledge that it is a huge struggle. Part of me wants to die and part of me doesn't . . . It was exhausting the struggle, but I gained strength as it went on.' (Int. N3)

'The PET helped me get in touch with what I needed to do with regard to grieving for my grand daughter.' (Int. S3) (implying that the suicide attempt was about that lack of grieving)

'I felt pushed at times, later in the process, but it kind of worked.' (Int. N3)

To conceptualize the key processes in this category, finding meaning in what may on the outside seem desperate rather than meaningful activity can help the suicidal people gain some power over their relationship with suicidality. Suicidality, to some extent, remains present, as an option in the suicidal person's life choices, and putting it in its place is a process rather than an epiphany. While the suicidality can remain present, by putting it 'in its place', the suicidal person can engage in more rational and informed choice when life becomes difficult. Previously, the suicidality was an apparent solution to the pain the suicidal person was experiencing, and as she/he understand the layers of suicidality, a more sophisticated analysis of suicidality becomes possible and, for some of the suicidal people in this study, it is defined as both a friend and a foe. When the suicidal person acknowledges the drastic and dramatic effects of the suicidality in the past (on self and others) it can act as a present and future deterrent. Managing the relationship with suicidality is hard work, and it is long term because the suicidality is ever present. The P/MH nurse helps with the emotional hard work by joining with the suicidal person to find the meaning of the suicide in the past/present/future.

Chapter 8

Theoretical Refutations and Practice Implications

'All our present well-meaning attention to demographic variables (age, sex ethnicity, etc.) and all our analysis of the ongoing electrochemical activities of the brain, cannot tell what we centrally want to know about the drama of emotions in the mind, the constricted thinking and the aching for peace.'
Shneidman 1997, p 29

CHAPTER CONTENTS

INTRODUCTION

It is often argued that nursing is a practice-based or practice-orientated discipline; for some (see Pearson 1992) practice is the *alpha and omega* of nursing and thus research undertaken for P/MH nursing should speak to and inform practice. Furthermore, a linked argument exists which purports that a hallmark of high quality P/MH nursing research is that the ensuing discussion considers the implications for practice that arise from the study findings (Cutcliffe & Ward 2006). Accordingly, we have identified seven distinct practice implications arising from the findings (theory) described in this book and these are summarized in Box 8.1. In keeping with Glaser and Strauss' (1967) and Glaser's (1978, 1992) position, the theory induced is a substantive grounded theory, in that its scope is that of the substantive area of care for the suicidal person. Consequently, it is prudent and necessary for the authors to discuss the implications of the findings in the context of that substantive area.

However, any such discussion is perhaps prefaced by a need to establish that the induced theory is robust. Normative approaches to discussions of research results require the researchers to compare the findings with existing empirical work; most often to indicate supporting evidence. The merits of this approach notwithstanding, we have adopted a Popperian approach (Popper 1965) in the sense that we attempt to refute the findings reported in this book through comparison with the extant empirical literature. Popper (1965) asserts that if researchers cannot 'disprove' their theory then this adds substantially to its credibility and authenticity. However, it should be noted that the authors are hindered in this endeavour since the width and depth of the extant literature is hardly extensive.

Nevertheless, this often-used method to gauge the robustness of the findings (theory) requires comparison with the existing literature and uses it as a 'conceptual mirror'. However, as the authors have already pointed out, there is only a very limited literature in this area. Therefore, the authors begin by first comparing the outcomes of this study with this limited literature; then they compare the findings from the study with related literatures, though not literature that has investigated the same issue. In other words, the findings of this study are first compared with the limited literature that has examined the experiences of being suicidal and the experiences of care during these times. The next comparison is with literature that refers to risk of suicide, particularly risk subsequent to discharge. The last comparison is with the literature that focuses on 'observations' as the principle approach for 'caring' for the suicidal person. Following this comparison, in order to include a thorough and comprehensive discussion, the implications for the theory will be considered in terms of the practice, research and policy issues.

Conceptual mirrors as a means to undertake theoretical refutation: comparison with the limited extant literature that has examined the experiences of being suicidal and the experiences of care during these times

Three papers/manuscripts relate to suicide from the individuals perspective, these are Walen (2002), Samuelsson et al (2000) and Crook (2003). It is particularly noticeable far from refuting the processes described in the three stages of our theory actually, many parallels exist between these and the limited literature. Each of the three stages of our theory will be considered in turn.

In stage one participants described a process of withdrawing from humanity. In her personal narrative about her life and suicide, Walen (2002, p 421) describes a powerful picture of her withdrawal from others. She likens this to that of being if in a void; she describes the loneliness as the most painful part of feeling suicidal. Similarly, Samuelsson et al (2000) reported that study participants felt isolated, yet ignored by ward staff. This suggests that despite withdrawing from all that about them, the suicidal people in this study were still aware of the need for human contact. Interestingly, our study findings note and emphasise the value of the intensive contact with the P/MH nurse, whereas Samulesson et al (2000) describes the nurses' reluctance to communicate with people in distress, due to lack of confidence in relating to such people. At first glance this might be taken as an example of refutation; closer consider however, perhaps indicates that this is not the case. In Samulesson's study, the P/MH nurses' reluctance to communicate did not bring about any therapeutic outcomes; indeed, this *de facto* disconnection only compounded the suicidal person's sense of isolation and disconnection. Interestingly, perhaps refutation of the findings reported in our study can be found in Crook's (2003) study, but at the same time, similarities are evident. Crook interviewed teenagers who had attempted suicide; she found that they wanted help but did not know where to look for it. Solace was sought from close friends who were prepared to sit and talk for many hours until some of the issues had been resolved and the crisis was less urgent. Thus, the findings in our study concerning the novel nature of the relationship formed between the P/MH and the suicidal person are not supported by Crook's study. What appears to be supported however, is (again) the value of re-connecting with humanity; in this case brought about (at least in part) by talking and being listened to (see stage one). Indeed, Walen (2002) postulates that, for the people in that study, talking through a problem helped take away the sense of constriction; helped the suicidal person move away from persistent suicidal thinking.

Further support rather than refutation exists in these three papers. In stage one of the theory described in this book, the authors highlighted how the environment, both internal to the person and the physical environment about them, can be 'manipulated' in order to help the person in suicidal distress. The participants in the study of Samuelsson et al (2000) noted the value (if not necessity) of being cared for in an atmosphere that is relaxing, welcoming, safe and friendly. A calming environment offers the chance for the individual to feel comfortable enough to talk about their experiences to the P/MH nurse.

The suicidal individuals in our study expressed the need to feel understood by P/MH nursing staff and the participants in the study of Samuelsson et al (2000) reported the same findings. In addition, Samulesson et al found that the action of showing the person that they are understood encourages feelings of hope to surface. Feeling cared about was repeatedly reported in the supporting literature (Crook 2003, Samuelsson et al 2002, Walen 2003). For Walen (2003) in particular, a timely demonstration of care from her psychiatrist prevented her from taking that last step towards ending her life.

In stage two of the theory described in this book, a re-connection with humanity was brought about (in part) by the suicidal person experiencing a particular and novel helping relationship with his/her P/MH nurse; this form of connection is not experienced in other spheres of the person's life. This finding did not appear to be supported by these three studies. Although it should be noted that while this 'special' relationship is not discussed explicitly in any of the supporting literature, Samuelsson et al (2000) do report that the most valued staff on the ward were trained P/MH nurses who were willing to engage with the individual.

There was clear support from these three papers rather than refutation of the findings in this study in relation to the suicidal person's moments of awareness regarding the implications of their suicide attempt on their own life and on those close to them. Samuelsson et al (2000), in particular, reported suicidal individuals as saying that they were shocked at what they had done and that this realization had prompted them to engage in a search for professional help. These same sentiments were found in the words of the participants in our study findings.

No references were found that related to the value of inner strength or personal beliefs in aiding the person's recovery from suicidality. However, both Crook (2003) and Samuelsson et al (2000) discuss the value of P/MH nurses bolstering the individual's self esteem. Walen (2003, p 428) is a strong advocate of the value of positive re-framing. She attributes much of her help to the 'unflagging optimism' on the part of her psychiatrist.

The findings in our study indicate that support was required for some time after the suicide attempt. Rather than refuting these findings, Samuelsson et al (2000) also found that study participants welcomed the offer to contact the ward at any time following discharge from hospital. Walen (2002) similarly supports the possibility that suicidal thoughts continue long after the person is considered to be 'well'. She purports that she continues to think about death on a regular basis, even though she also states that she is happier than she has ever been before in her life. However, she also notes that thinking about suicide provides a comforting option to her. Contemplating suicide, she says, takes up much energy, which might be an effective way of keeping ones self from enacting it. Participants in this study talked of their continuing relationship with suicide also.

In summary, although there is very little literature with which to compare and contrast the findings of this study, what is available contains some strong similarities and appears to lend credibility, rather than refute the views that the theory induced from this study is robust.

Conceptual mirrors as a means to undertake theoretical refutation: comparison with the extant literature that refers to risk of suicide subsequent to discharge

There is a wealth of literature that focuses on risk of suicide, identifying risk factors, calculating risk factors, determining interactions between risk factors and risk factors as predictors of suicide. Indeed, this may be the largest discrete body of literature that relates to suicide. A sub-category of this body of literature is that which considers risk after discharge, or to rephrase, the continuing presence and estimation of risk of suicide following intervention from formal healthcare services. It is noteworthy that this is a less substantial literature. This is perhaps rather counter-intuitive given that we do know that one of the most reliable predictors of a future suicide attempt is a previous suicide attempt. Nevertheless, there is a body of literature that shows there is a distinct difference between the rates of suicide for those people recently discharged from psychiatric services compared to the average rates for the male/female population.

The significantly increased risk of suicide following discharge from an inpatient psychiatric service has been shown in a number of studies (see for example, Geddes & Juszczak 1995, Geddes et al 1997, Goldacre et al 1993, Roy 1982). In a study focusing on the population of the Oxford health region of the UK, Goldacre et al (1993) calculated the standardized mortality ratio (SMR) for suicide in the first 28 days following discharge from inpatient psychiatric services. Starting from the premise that the SMR value for the 'general population' is 1, they calculated that the SMR for male completed suicides was 213 (95% Confidence Interval{CI} 137–317) and for females the SMR was 134 (95% CI, 67–240). More alarmingly, additional calculations undertaken by Goldacre et al (1993) indicated that the period of time immediately following discharge was the highest risk time. The suicide rate in the first 28 days following discharge was 7.1 (95% CI, 4.1–12) times higher for male patients and 3.0 (95% CI, 1.5–6.0) times higher for female patients than the rate in the subsequent later 48 weeks of the first year after discharge from psychiatric inpatient care. Such increased risk is by no means isolated to the United Kingdom as the study undertaken by Ho (2003) demonstrates. Using a similar method and design to Goldacre et al, Ho examined the suicide rates of recently discharged psychiatric patients from psychiatric hospitals in Hong Kong. In the first 28 days following discharge, the SMR for males was 113 (95% CI, 86–147) and for females was 178 (95% CI, 132–235). (Again, using the general population rate as 1.) The rates in the first 28 days versus 29–365 days were 4.6 times higher in males and 4 times higher in females. Indeed, the evidence in this study indicated that between 16 and 38% of all suicides within the year following discharge occurred in the first month (Ho 2003). Thus, the magnitude of risk following discharge was similar in both studies.

Additional studies have produced very similar findings. Geddes et al (1997), for example, also used a similar method and design to Goldacre et al to examine suicide rates in recently discharged psychiatric patients in Scotland from 1968 to 1992. Although they found a significant increase in the risk of suicide in the first 28 days versus the rest of the first year following discharge, the ratio of 1–28 to 29–365 days was 1.7 (95% CI, 1.4–1.9) for males and 1.6 (95% CI, 1.3–1.8) for females. More recently, in a related study, Hawton et al (2003) studied the risk of suicide for those people who present to hospital services. Somewhat alarmingly, they found that such people have a considerable risk to die as a result of suicide in the first year following the attempt; indeed their level of risk was calculated to be 66 times the annual risk in the general population. The 1996 Confidential Inquiry into Deaths by Suicide in Sheffield (Dickinson et al 1996) indicated that almost 30% of identified completed suicides had been under psychiatric care in the recent past, findings echoed by the more comprehensive National Confidential Inquiry described previously. The findings therein indicated that 23, 26 and 30% of the suicides in England, Scotland and Northern Ireland died within 3 months of discharge from psychiatric care. Post-discharge suicides were at a peak 1–2 weeks following discharge.

Two recent studies have continued to document the high proportion of suicides in the first months following discharge. King et al (2001) studied all suicides and open verdicts given to residents of Hampshire, Dorset, Wiltshire and the Isle of Wight during the years 1988–1997. They located 373 suicides/open verdicts of individuals who died before discharge or within a year of discharge from a psychiatric inpatient stay. Of this total, 298 patients died following discharge and 34% (of 234 cases that met the inclusion criteria) of these discharged patients suicided within 28 days of discharge and 61% suicided within 3 months of discharge. Robinson and colleagues (Robinson et al 2002) published an abstract based on The National Clinical Survey which is a survey of all suicides of individuals with mental health service contact in the year before their death in the UK. Of all the suicides, 5099 suicides (24% of all reported suicides) had contact with Mental Health Services and data was available on 4859 of these suicides. The suicides tended to cluster in the first week or around discharge from hospital with 23% of the suicides occurring within 3 months of discharge. Qin and Nordentoft (2005) calculated the population attributable risk based on their findings from Danish national longitudinal registers and estimated that prevention efforts during the first week after discharge might impact up to 2.1% of male and 3.8% of female suicides.

It is difficult to ignore the compelling nature of this epidemiological evidence, and not surprisingly, it has led to a number of explanations for the increased risk following discharge. The high risk of suicide has been attributed to either the lack of improvement of patients during their admission or failures in the continuity of care following discharge. In Morgan and Priest's (1991) study of the 27 psychiatric in-patients who committed suicide (either during their hospitalization or during the 3 months immediately following discharge), suicide risk had been discussed, but in only 10 cases had any precautions been introduced. This suggested that some people who felt suicidal post-discharge were undetected and, for 17 people in the sample, the suicide risk appeared to be underestimated.

McKenzie and Wurr (2001) examined predictors of early suicide following discharge from a psychiatric hospital and found that the early suicides versus the non-suicidal subjects were significantly more likely to have a past history of deliberate self-harm, a diagnosis of mood disorder and longer case records that implied that their last admissions to hospital were more complicated that the comparison groups' admissions. King et al (2001) used a case-control design to study risk factors for patient suicides following discharge and identified eleven factors that were associated with an increased risk of suicide following discharge. The factor, 'key personnel on leave' was related to a 16-fold increased risk of suicide and was in keeping with the explanation that lack of continuity of care might be an important causal factor. Also supportive of the continuity model was the intervention trial by Motto and Bostrom (2001). They demonstrated that the simple contact by letter, suggesting the importance of 'connectiveness', following discharge from hospital was sufficient to reduce the risk of suicide after discharge. Our current limited understanding leads Hoyer et al (2004, p 215) to note that: 'At admission, the patients are acutely ill and maybe suicidal, but we do not have any explanation for the high risk of suicide immediately after discharge.'

Morgan (1994) offers a tentative explanation for this post-discharge high risk of suicide. He argues that decisions to discharge former suicidal clients should not be based on symptomatic improvement. He purports that unless the person's situational and precipitating events factors are dealt with effectively, there is a risk of catastrophic 'relapse' following discharge, and thus in these circumstances, the risk of suicide following discharge is high.

In an attempt to deepen our understanding of this post-discharge risk of suicide, and the linked issue of contact as a means to enhance connectedness, two studies should be noted, Welu (1977) and Motto and Bostrom (2001). Welu's (1977) study makes the case (the methodological limitations of the study not withstanding) that the more intense follow up a 'formerly suicidal' person receives post-discharge, the higher the positive correlation with reduced attempts. Similarly, Motto and Bostrom's (2001) study provides illuminating evidence. In their study a total of 843 discharged clients were divided into two groups. The independent variable group ('contact' group) received contact at least four times a year for the next 5 years; the control group received no contact. Clients in the contact group had a lower suicide rate in all 5 years. More noticeably, the survival analysis revealed a significantly lower rate in the contact group during the first 2 years following discharge. Differences in the rate gradually diminished and by year 14 no differences were observed between the groups.

As a result of comparing the epidemiological evidence and the tentative theoretical explanations above with the findings from our study, rather than refute our findings, there is clear support. In stage three of our theory, we explained how the participants in our study had engaged in the process of making sense of their suicidal act. Further, that this 'sense making' was being achieved through an array of interpersonal processes, including supportive involvement from professionals (mainly P/MH nurses in this study), family and fellow travellers on the suicidality path. The research participants also alluded to how dealing with their existential angst was no easy task; it was taking time and effort. Learning how to go on living again, but now with the suicide act as part of their tapestry of experience was thus something that the participants were aware of; and they were aware that this was unlikely to be resolved quickly. Thus while, in the view of the formal psychiatric services, the participants had passed their 'acute, suicidal crisis', from the participants' perspective, there was still significant work to be done. It is perhaps then not altogether surprising that there is risk of suicide post-discharge if one accepts the findings in our study that the 'meaning making' work remains incomplete. While the authors would in no way wish to purport that this theory can account for or explain all post-discharge risk of suicide, we do believe that this theory offers one possible explanation and it is worthy of further consideration and study.

Conceptual mirrors as a means to undertake theoretical refutation: comparison with the extant 'Observation' literature

There is a substantive extant literature that focuses on 'observations' and posits these as the principal *modus operandi* for providing 'care' to the suicidal person. Indeed, some of this has already been covered and discussed in Chapter 2. The authors have no desire to pointlessly repeat themselves, but there is merit in re-asserting some of the principal features of this literature and then comparing these with our findings.

It is important to re-state that no clinical controlled trials have yet been undertaken to determine whether or not observation does in fact keep suicidal people safe, let alone whether or not it helps suicidal people deal with their psychache, their hopelessness and their suicidal thoughts. The basic premise that would form the basis for refuting our findings might be: if observations (or whatever vernacular term is used to describe this practice) are shown to be effective and our theory suggests otherwise, then the observation literature can be used to refute our findings.

Yet, the limited literature we do have can hardly be regarded as providing a cogent case for indicating and supporting the efficacy of observations as a means to care for suicidal people. The Department of Health (2001) Safety First report highlighted that *18% of all completed mental health inpatient suicides occurred while people were under observation* (our emphasis). Other studies and audits (see for example, Cutcliffe and Ramcharan 2002) have repeatedly shown that many completed suicides continue to occur while people were 'under' observation. Further, despite the as yet untested protestations of some (see for example Bowers 2001), there has been no exponential increase in suicide when observations was replaced (see Bowles et al 2002, Dodds & Bowles 2001). Also, in the study which is often touted as providing 'supportive evidence' for the case of observations (Cardell & Pitula 1999), a more discerning examination of these findings shows that it is not being under observations *per se* that helps suicidal people, but the experience of being engaged with during such time. Alarmingly, this study also provides evidence that being 'under observations' can actually cause the suicidal person to deliberately mislead those observing him/her as a means to end the ordeal of being observed. In keeping with Cardell and Pitula's study, other evidence pertaining to the experience(s) of being observed is equivocal, though there appears to be a trend towards service users expressing more criticisms than support (see for example, Barker and Walker 1999, Bowles et al 2002, Fletcher 1999, Jones et al 2000).

There appears to be widespread consensus within this debate that caring for suicidal people is a complicated, difficult and challenging task that requires highly educated and trained practitioners. Yet, the same consensus shows that, in the large majority of cases, this care is not provided by such individuals; quite the contrary. International evidence repeatedly shows that observations are carried out by non-psychiatric nurses; indeed there is a discernable trend towards the use of sitters, security guards, and closed-circuit TV cameras (see for example, Cardell & Pitula 1999, Cutcliffe 2002, Holmes et al 2004, Jones & Jackson 2004, Ward & Jones 2006). Despite the claims of those whom would advocate for the use of observations in the care of suicidal people, the evidence is largely consistent in showing that it is more and more used entirely and solely as a defensive practice.

In summary of this section, there is a substantial literature that relates to observations and the care of suicidal people, though very little empirical work exists. What literature is available cannot be seen to constitute a compelling case for the efficacy of observations as a means to care for suicidal people – on the contrary. The existing literature also clearly shows a movement towards observations as a low-skill activity carried out by non-psychiatric nurses and in the worse cases, carried out through a closed circuit TV camera and thus there is no human contact whatsoever. Such findings cannot be regarded to constitute a robust argument that refutes the findings and result views emerging from the findings in our study.

PRACTICE IMPLICATIONS

As stated above, there are a number of practice implications arising out of this study; these are listed, in no specific order of priority in Box 8.1, and then each is discussed in detail.

Practice discussion point one: P/MH nurses need to be comfortable with death – talking about suicide

Few credible P/MH nurses would disagree that their practice is essentially an interpersonal endeavour; one that is inherently concerned with listening and talking. According to the findings in our study, P/MH nurses need to be comfortable with co-presencing; to be able to sit with the suicidal patients' and the P/MH nurses' own emotions that surround the experience(s) of death, suicide and mortality. While some P/MH nurses may feel that they are already comfortable with this (and that may very well be the case), there is a body of evidence that shows how for many, dealing with emotionally charged experiences such as death and suicide is often problematic and is sometimes avoided altogether. Evidence of this dynamic is evident in both seminal and more contemporary literature.

Box 8.1 Practice discussion points

1. P/MH nurses need to be comfortable with death – talking about suicide.
2. P/MH nurse's need to be comfortable with co-presencing; they need to learn to 'talk to listen' not 'listen to talk'.
3. Additional education/training in order to provide care for/with the suicidal person is necessary.
4. Observation needs to be replaced with engagement.
5. P/MH nurses need to move away from models of care for the suicidal person that focus and rely on 'medication based' work and instead, focus on 'interpersonal based' work.
6. P/MH nurses (and other formal mental health professionals) need to move away from 'risk focused' work to 'care focused' work and undertake a radical shift in conceptualizations of what constitutes an appropriate time frame for care of the suicidal person.
7. P/MH nursing care for the suicidal person needs to be based in a 'recovery' and not a 'cure' model.

In the UK, Professor Annie Altschul was attuned to the importance of inter-personal relations as the foundation of effective P/MH nursing. She studied nurse–patient interactions and arrived at the conclusion that P/MH nurses largely shunned any contact with patients (Altschul 1972), consistently spending their time in the office and only c. 10% with patients. Altschul's conclusions about psychiatric nursing are an echo of the earlier work of Menzies (1959, 1961) in relation to 'general' nurses' response to suffering and death. Menzies drew on the psychodynamic work of Melanie Klein and in so doing argued that nurses use 'ego defence mechanisms' in order to prevent anxiety provoked by emotionally intense situations with patients. Such anxiety arises because the nurse has her own inner fantasy world, constructed during infancy, in which the child, and people with whom the child is tied emotionally, play out different relationships. Because of the aggressive forces within the child, many of the fantasies are negative or destructive. 'Unconsciously, the nurse associates the patient's and relatives' distress with that experienced by the people in her fantasy world, which increases her own anxiety and difficulty in handling it' (Menzies-Lyth 1988, p 48). More recently, Sanon-Rollins (2006) drew attention to the survey made of three hospitals. The findings revealed that regardless of institutional or demographic characteristics, nurses use avoidance as a primary strategy to resolve conflict, including their own internal conflict.

Even more cursory examination of the bereavement counselling literature will show that dealing with the issues or topics of death and dying often provokes feelings of discomfort in the listener. Accordingly, it is not surprisingly that some nurses still have significant discomfort when talking about situations which are synonymous with death and dying. Coupled with these emotionally charged issues is the qualitatively different nature of death (or attempted death) by suicide (see Chapter 10 for a more thorough discussion on this matter). Yet, as the findings in our study indicate, it was imperative for the P/MH nurse to be able to be with the suicidal person and listen intently to highly personalized accounts of suicide and suicidality. Without so doing, the process of re-connecting would be hindered if not actually thwarted.

Thus, P/MH nurses working with a person who has made a serious suicidal attempt need to be thoroughly prepared to hear about death, dying and suicide and moreover, not shy away from this; not be uncomfortable with the topic(s) nor discourage the suicidal person from talking openly about his/her suicidality and psychache. A similar argument has been postulated previously by Davidhizar and Vance (1993) who also stressed that when working with suicidal people, P/MH nurses need to consider their own attitudes towards suicide in order that they can ensure they do not distance themselves from the suicidal person. Such consideration clearly demands and requires that the P/MH nurse needs to possess a high degree of self-awareness; and needs to have come to terms with his/her own mortality.

Practice discussion point two: P/MH nurse's need to be comfortable with co-presencing; they need to learn to 'talk to listen' not 'listen to talk'

Following on from the previous practice discussion point, and clearly also linked to that, is the need for P/MH nurses to be able to co-presence and listen. All too often and for a variety of reasons, some nurses are too quick to speak.

Sometimes, nurses have a compelling need to be seen to be doing; to be active; to be making a difference. Sometimes, nurses use their own talk as a defence mechanism; if the nurse is talking the majority of the time it is difficult for the suicidal person to bring up emotive (and dangerous) issues. Sometimes, with every good intent, some nurses wish to find the erudite sentence; the 'pearl of wisdom' that will serve as an epiphany and solve all the suicidal person's problems in one go.

Yet, sometimes the hardest thing to do is nothing! While this truism is used here purposefully to make the point, it should not detract from the message the authors are trying to make. The suicidal people in this study welcomed the chance to talk and be heard; to speak and be understood and to gain a sense that somebody cared. This was brought about (in part) by the P/MH nurse saying little and hearing a lot. The authors will not belabour the link between the first two discussion points, but the P/MH nurse's willingness to really listen to the suicidal client is clearly prefaced by the P/MH nurse's high degree of comfort in hearing such disclosures. If the P/MH nurse is unable or unwilling to hear about the person's suicidality, then he/she is unlikely to listen.

For the suicidal person recovering her/his life force, it is critical to have space in which to make sense of what has happened to her/him. To some extent, this work takes place in the private domain, but the involvement of the P/MH was pivotal to the participants of this study. The P/MH nurses asked questions that encouraged the outward expression of ideas, hopes and fears and then demonstrated the capacity to listen to the suicidal person's innermost concerns; they were able to ask 'Where does it hurt?' and subsequently, hear the person's story. This process encourages a sense of co-presence for the suicidal person.

Furthermore, the findings in this study illustrate the importance of P/MH nurses being able to hold back from being too instrumental too soon. In other words, P/MH nurses must be able to judge the pace that the suicidal person needs to travel at. Peplau (1952) believed that the P/MH nurse needs to be sensitive to the patient's needs at different times and adopt a role of 'friend' or 'teacher' or 'parental figure', etc., accordingly. Similarly, Jackson and Stevenson (2000) supported Peplau's findings almost 50 years later in a study which asked: 'What do people need psychiatric and mental health nurses for?'. In their study, a grounded theory was inducted based on the perceptions of the care process of service users, carers, P/MH nurses and multidisciplinary colleagues. The theory identified the fluctuating degree of friendliness versus professional intervention present within the nurse–client relationship. This needed to be judged by the P/MH nurse on the basis of cues provided by the person as service user. As a result, there was a time for being more instrumental and a time for being less instrumental; findings that clearly resonate with the findings reported in this book.

Practice discussion point three: Additional education/training in how to provide care for/with the suicidal person is necessary

One of the more common features of research reports it seems is the inclusion of 'standard recommendations' whereby authors inevitably highlight the need for:

(a) more research and,
(b) additional training/education of practitioners is indicated.

These are laudable and often appropriate recommendations, but in the view of the current authors, perhaps such recommendations lack specificity and precision. This is especially the case if one accepts the axiom that good research should generate more questions than it answers (hence the need for more research) and that research should inform practice (and thus the need for additional education/training for practitioners). Consequently, it is not without serious consideration that the authors include recommendation three here. However, the findings were so compelling in the face of the current customs and practice of many formal care settings for care of the suicidal person that it would be remiss of the authors not to include such a recommendation.

The findings in our study indicated the presence of a good practice. Interestingly, even the P/MH nurses in our study who demonstrated this good practice had received little or no formal education or training for care of the suicidal person. Their skills had been picked up over their many years of experience. While there is nothing inherently wrong with such experiential ('on the job') training, we know that such training will include making mistakes. Indeed, some might argue that this is an inherent aspect of experiential learning. Furthermore, the situation that P/MH nurses should need to care for suicidal people without having had any specific training is unacceptable; particularly in the face of the compelling evidence already highlighted in this book regarding suicide and people with mental health problems. In the recent National Confidential Inquiry into Homicides and Suicides, (Department of Health 1999b, 2001) it was indicted that approximately one quarter of the people who took their own lives in England and Wales, Scotland and Northern Ireland had been in contact with mental health services in the year before death. The report indicates that 16% of the reported suicide cases in England, Wales, 12% in Scotland and 10.5% in Northern Ireland were psychiatric patients. Of particular note, many of the practitioners contacted in the inquiry felt that many of the suicides could have been avoided. This epidemiological and 'clinical' picture is echoed in many countries from around the world (see Chapters 1 and 2).

It is worth looking at the current situation regarding preparation of P/MH nurses and more specifically, preparing these practitioners to work with suicidal people. P/MH nursing curricula, whether pre or post-graduation, almost inevitably make reference (to a greater or lesser extent) to suicide. Differences are common and not surprising between specialist and generic pre-registration curricula. Restricted by constraints of time and space, and by the demands of competing areas of care/issues for nurses, generic programmes often have less attention to suicide (and still less devoted to care of the suicidal person) than specialist programmes. The diminution of specialisms within generic programmes is inevitable. Chan and Rudman (1998, p 144), purport: 'the tendency towards the majority (in nurse education) invariably produces distortion at the expense of academic rigor in the specialities.'

Yet, specialist P/MH programmes have no place for complacency and arguably are still severely limited in their preparing P/MH to care for suicidal people. Almost inevitably, the focus in such curricula is an introduction to the principal theories of suicide (rightly so) and then material on risk and risk assessment; very little attention is given to what P/MH nurses might do by way of caring for suicidal people once the risk assessment is complete (other than perhaps assigning and instigating various forms of defensive practice and administering medication). In no way are the authors of this paper wishing to decry and diminish the value and necessity of thorough and accurate risk assessment; these are invaluable skills and must remain as part of P/MH nursing curricula. Risk assessment though is only one component of the larger whole; it is not an end in and of itself. P/MH nursing curricula need to evolve to include options, strategies, interventions and a variety of theoretical approaches in order to equip P/MH with a range of skills, knowledge and attitudes required for providing effective care to suicidal people. However, it would be inappropriate to admonish the designers of these curricula for omitting material regarding interventions, even more so evidence-based interventions, given the paucity of tested and efficacious interventions that exist. Indeed, one of the most pressing needs of the international suicidology academe, including P/MH nurses, is to produce a range of workable, theoretically robust and evidence-based interventions for working with suicidal people.

It may well be, as with other specialist areas of practice, that the best we can achieve in basic P/MH education is to equip students with risk assessment skills, familiarity with suicide risk tools, some intervention skills such as active listening, personal awareness raising of their own issues around death, dying and suicide, and the beginnings of the development of the required qualities. It may well be that additional specialist, advanced education and training would be required for those P/MH nurses who wish to focus on working with suicidal people. Just as we would not expect newly graduated P/MH nurses to take on a caseload of people requiring specialist psychotherapy, the authors suggest it would be clinically prudent not to expect newly graduated P/MH nurses to take on a case load 'heavy' with highly suicidal people. This appears to be particularly logical and sensible given the previously mentioned complexity of suicide and the emotional requirements such clients demand of their P/MH nurses.

It is interesting to note that most often the exhortations contained with inquiries following mental health inpatient suicide deaths and the ensuing various well-meaning publications (see for example Jones & Jackson 2004), the only additional training or education advocated for is further 'refresher' courses for carrying out observations and others calling for more training is risk assessment. Lastly, though it is not a finding directly related to P/MH nursing, the problem of inadequate preparation for caring for suicidal people was highlighted in Egan's (1997) study. That survey of 112 psychiatrists and psychologists revealed that most had never received formal training in the implementation of no-suicide contracts for patients at risk of suicide.

Consequently, it is evident that both the current preparation of P/MH nurses to work with suicidal people, and the extant formal psychiatric and mental healthcare system is deficient in providing adequate, therapeutic, transformative care for suicidal people. It is also evident that the practitioners themselves recognize the deficiencies in the system, and these are echoed in the findings in this study. Participants in this study spoke clearly of the difficulties they had coming to terms with their suicidal act and their suicidal episode. What became evident, and this is something that the services did not appear to account for, was the need for longer term input and therapeutic work for suicidal clients. Essentially, these people reported needing additional help from the formal mental health care services with making sense of their suicide act/episode. How these people 'wove' this experience into the 'tapestry' of their life was not clear, but it was clear that this process often took more time than the formal mental health services offered to the people. Hence, there is a clear need to provide additional education/training to address this matter.

In addition to providing the training that would increase the practitioner's awareness of a longer 'care episode' for suicidal clients, is the parallel need for additional education for the day to day, minute to minute care. As stated above, P/MH nurses need to be comfortable with co-presencing, to be able to sit with both the patients' and their own emotions that surround the near experience of death. All too often, some practitioners have either prejudicial attitudes towards suicide (and thus the suicidal person), or are uncomfortable with suicide; often feeling that they lack the 'right words to say'. Consequently, there is a clear need to engage in self-awareness raising training, particularly around attitudes towards suicide, death and one's own mortality. There is a need for practitioners to learn how to be comfortable with expressions of death, to learn how to be comfortable with suicidal or 'death orientated' people despite not having 'pat' phrases or clever answers.

Practice discussion point four: 'Observations' needs to be replaced with 'Engagement'

One of the first things that becomes evident upon examining the extant P/MH nursing suicide related literature is that this is currently an area of 'care' that is synonymous with 'defensive practices'. Defensive practices, in this instance, are those concerned (to a greater or lesser extent) with the following issues:

1. They are concerned with meeting the needs of the organization.
2. They are concerned with preventing a person from causing physical harm to himself or herself.
3. They serve the need of avoiding, off-setting or 'side-stepping' potential litigation.
4. They are concerned with the physical integrity of the person and do little (or nothing) to address the genesis (and/or exacerbation) of the person's suicidal thoughts or feelings.
5. They provide little (or nothing) in the way of addressing, relieving or helping the suicidal person's 'psychache' (Shneidman 1997), or pervasive sense of hopelessness (Weishaar 2000) and thus do little (or nothing) to address the emotional, psychological or spiritual needs and well-being of the suicidal person (see Barker & Cutcliffe 1999, Bowles et al 2002, Cutcliffe & Barker 2002, Dodds & Bowles 2001).

In the context of care for the suicidal person, these defensive practices include, or perhaps more accurately, are epitomized by 'close observations' (or whatever vernacular term is used in different countries, e.g. specialling, 'one-to-one's', arms length observations) and to a lesser extent by seclusion rooms, physical restraints, and closed-circuit TV monitoring. Recent examples of this emphasis on defensive practices for care of the suicidal person can be seen in the United Kingdom's Standing Nursing and Midwifery Advisory

Committee's (1999) practice guidelines for 'safe and supportive' observations of the mental health client at risk of harming him or herself. Additional emphasis can be found in the recommendations of the largest (and most expensive) review of suicide deaths of people with mental health problems, the National Confidential Inquiry (Department of Health 2001). The 1999 guidelines list 12 recommendations for carrying out observations and the only reference to working with the person's suicidal ideation and/or feelings is perhaps the oblique statement: 'Every effort should be made to promote a therapeutic relationship with the patient; minimizing the distress caused by the process (of being observed).' Even this laudable endeavor says nothing about helping the person with their suicidal thoughts/feelings and further it is noteworthy that of the 12 guidelines, this in number eight.

Similarly, the clear emphasis of the recommendations contained within the 'Safety First' (Department of Health 2001) document was the tightening up of current observations policies, additional attention to the transfer of clients from one agency to another and greater control of the physical environment as an effort to decrease the availability for people to have means to harm themselves. Accordingly, the recommendation to install collapsible curtain rails around the client's 'bed-space' should be used in order to prevent clients from having a ligature point.

These environmental focused defensive interventions may have utility, and they have some empirical support (Department of Health 2005). However, it is worth noting the evidence related to previous 'environmental' focused interventions. Perhaps the best example of this occurred when attempts were made to reduce the suicide rate in the general population by changing the household gas supplies from a toxic to a non-toxic gas. While there was a corresponding drop in suicide rates (particularly for women and housewives) (Dunnell 1994), unfortunately, the longitudinal data indicated the rates began to increase again once alternative methods were 'discovered'. Accordingly, while there may be limited utility in such environmental related, defensive practices, the long-term efficacy is questionable and clearly on their own, such interventions are not the answer to helping suicidal people.

Now, these defensive practices described above need to be considered in the context of the following axioms:

Axiom 1: suicide is a complex, convoluted, multi-dimensional problem

The international suicidology academe is in agreement that suicide is a complex, multi-dimensional phenomenon and yet our understanding of it is far from complete (see for example, Canadian Association for Suicide Prevention 2004, Leenaars 2004, Maris 1997a). It belies attempts to simplify or define the phenomenon (Leenaars 2004). It transcends the barriers of a 'health' and 'social' problem and thus results in, what former President of the American Association of Suicidology, Rod Maris terms the biopsychosocial perspective of suicide (Maris 1997a). This complexity is captured by Maris when he states: 'Because suicide is not one kind of behavior, the explanation of suicide cannot be by a single factor or the province solely of any one professional discipline or specialty area' (Maris 1997a, p 53).

Axiom 2: observation as a means to 'treat' a person's suicidality has little or no empirical evidence to support it; there exists empirical evidence which shows that it fails in its principal function, i.e. keeping people physically safe, and more and more is carried out by workers who have no formal psychiatric nurse education or training

While it would be epistemologically premature to posit a simple causative relationship between high rates of suicide and high rates of defensive practice, it is hard to ignore the empirical and anecdotal evidence which we have included previously, that strongly suggests that defensive practices have, at best, a limited usefulness (and efficacy) in providing care to the suicidal person. Even if we were to invoke simplistic forms of logic, it would appear to be counter-intuitive (and an ill-advised choice) to 'treat' or 'care for' people with sophisticated, complex, multi-dimensional problems by preventing the physical means of attempting suicide, and hoping that the suicidal person spontaneously resolves whatever problems (and psychache) that ushered them towards suicide in the first instance. The extant literature is clear in highlighting the deficiencies of 'observations' and as a result, more sophisticated and less defensive forms of practice are needed to care for suicidal people.

With this in mind, the findings of our study clearly indicate that P/MH nurses need to develop different ways of relating to people who have an acquaintance with suicide. Currently, there is ample evidence within the literature to indicate that often people are held at arm's length emotionally while they are kept physically close. Often, such physical proximity, particularly without any attempt to address the person's emotional/psychological needs, is experienced as intrusive and unhelpful. Yet the evidence in this study clearly indicates that close observations were largely ineffectual in bringing about a re-connection with humanity. Indeed, in the cases where care of the suicidal person occurred in the community (majority of the cases), observations played little or (mostly) no part in the care. Consequently, despite the proliferation of policy literature that emphasizes observations and custodial care for the suicidal person (see for example the Standing Nursing and Midwifery Advisory Committee 1999), there is a need to abandon observations for care of the suicidal person as a matter of urgency. P/MH nurses need to make themselves available to suicidal people, albeit in a way that respects the pace that such people are comfortable with and which establishes a mutual engagement. The evidence, as shown earlier in this book, is consistent in showing that despite tighter 'policing' observation policies, people with mental health problems still take their own lives either during the periods of observation, when the observations are removed or soon after discharge. The findings in this study add to the case for abandoning observations by showing that suicidal people clearly benefit from a more 'engagement' focused model of care; one that attempts to address the genesis and experience of the whole suicidal episode rather than focusing on unsophisticated 'policing' of suicidal people.

Practice discussion point five: P/MH nurses need to move away from models of care for the suicidal person that rely and focus on 'medication' based work and instead, need to focus on interpersonal based work

P/MH nurses have sometimes had a difficult time in articulating what they do (Altschul 1997, Brown & Fowler 1979, Hill & Michael 1996). One thing that many P/MH nurses do become involved in and can articulate is the administering of medications and the subsequent monitoring of the effects/side-effects. Indeed, recent 'developments' in some countries have included giving limited powers of prescription to P/MH nurses. While it falls outside the scope of this book to include a full debate on that issue, and we include a more thorough discussion in chapter ten, the authors believe there is utility in examining if/how the findings from our study 'speak to' these issues.

The findings from our study cast more doubt on the (for some) automatically assumed value of psychotropic medications as the focus of care for the suicidal person. One of the most startling findings for the authors in this study was the shortness of the length of the 'suicide crisis'. It is important that the parameters of the care episode are understood here because they have significant implications. The participants in this study described how they had a 'crisis' period. This was, not surprisingly, matched with the most intensive input from the formal psychiatric services and consequently precipitated the intervention of the psychiatric emergency teams. What we then saw was a very short episode of intensive intervention. This was a matter of days. Crucially, the evidence provided by the participants tells us that they still had a distinct need for additional input in to 'make sense of' and 'find the meaning in' the suicide episode. However, the immediate crisis had been alleviated, most often over the period of a few days. In explaining the processes and dynamics of this significant 'change of heart' it cannot be ignored that anti-depressant medication needs two/three weeks before any major therapeutic effects will occur (Issacson & Rich 1997, Maris et al 2000). Thus, it would seem to be inappropriate and inaccurate to assign these dramatic 'changes of heart' that occurred with the participants in this study to the pharmaceutical action of anti-depressant medication. These findings echo those of Gunnell and Frankel (1994) who pointed out that several retrospective reviews of the treatments received by psychiatric patients provided no consistent evidence that anti-depressant medication reduced the likelihood of suicide. Indeed, Maris et al (2000, p 525) declare: 'Psychopharmacotherapy does not target suicide *per se*. There simply is no anti-suicide pill'.

Furthermore, the evidence from the participants in our study concerning the effectiveness and experience of taking medication was equivocal. As described in the category 'Recognizing the limits and value of pharmacological intervention' participants often spoke of their dissatisfaction with a variety of medications, and/or those with anxiolytic effects, their discomfort and dissatisfaction that all the healthcare services (at times) had to offer was 'another pill', and their discomfort with side-effects. Yet, there was also some evidence that indicated the therapeutic benefits and value that some people experienced as a result of taking some medications. (Notably, this tended to be short-term use of anxiolytic medications to give people a chance to sleep and a chance to experience a calmer period.) Even in these cases, though, focused and intensive interpersonal work occurred alongside any pharmacological intervention. While the medications may have created a temporary sense of calm, there remained a great deal of work to be done around the person's feelings/thoughts about being disconnected from humanity. The medication did not reconnect anyone, it (at times) provided a short period of respite, and in some cases, added to the sense of disconnection.

This evidence further challenges and contradicts current 'medication' based models for care of the suicidal person. This is not to suggest that there is no role or place for medication in the care of the suicidal person. But what it does do is locate the use of medication as an adjunct to the more appropriate interpersonal work. Furthermore, it clearly indicates where and what P/MH nurses might be principally concerned with in terms of providing care to suicidal people; for the person in suicidal crisis, the principal focus of work must be the interpersonal rather than pharmacological.

If one accepts the body of evidence that casts doubt on the utility of, and P/MH nurse's role in pharmacological intervention for suicidal people, and at the same time, the undeniable fact that suicide is a *human drama,* played out in the everyday lives, minds, brains and interactions of people, it may not be entirely surprising that, for P/MH nurses at any rate, caring for suicidal people must be an interpersonal endeavour; and one personified by talking and listening. As he does so often, Shneidman (1997, p 29) eloquently captures the essence of this message when he states:

> 'There is a basic rule to keep in mind: We can reduce the lethality if we lessen the anguish, the perturbation. Suicidal individuals who are asked, 'Where do you hurt?' intuitively know that this is a question about their emotions and their lives, and they answer appropriately, not in biological terms but with some literary or humanistic sophistication, in psychological terms. What I mean by this is to ask about the person's feelings, worries and pain.'

Views highly congruent with Shneidman's are expressed by Maltsberger (1992, cited in Maris et al 2000, p 13) when he asserts:

> 'As important as the biological treatment of hopelessness is, any treatment of a suicidal patient that relies solely on impersonal therapies (e.g. psychoactive medication, seclusion, restraint, and 15 minute checks (observations) may be second rate . . . Many psychiatrists argue that the heart of the treatment of suicidal individuals is the relationship of the therapists and the patient.'

Practice discussion point six: P/MH nurses (and other formal mental health professionals) need to move away from 'risk focused' work to 'care focused' work and undertake a radical shift in their conceptualizations of what constitutes an appropriate time frame for care of the suicidal person

As we have stated earlier in this book, one area of the extant suicidology literature that appears to be reasonably well developed is that of risk assessment, risk factors and risk management. The authors need to preface this discussion point by stating that we add our own exhortation to those already in existence that highlight the necessity and value of the most accurate assessment of risk possible. However, determining the degree of risk of suicide in a person is, arguably, only the beginning. Thorough and accurate risk assessment that does not lead to intervention is not only inadequate but a pathway to frustration. In order to emphasize this point, the authors would like to draw on the analogy of coronary care and the risk of myocardial infarction.

A significant and very well developed literature exists around the issue of risk factors in coronary care. Many of these are well known to members of the public; in no way are they restricted to the purview of medicine or healthcare. Several risk assessment tools have been developed and have shown to be reliable and valid. But where coronary care risk assessment differs markedly for assessing risk of suicide is that the assessment actually leads somewhere. Having undertaken the risk assessment a variety of primary, secondary and tertiary interventions are enacted. The person's diet is changed, exercise regimens are put in place, a variety of efficacious medications are prescribed and administered, family histories are explored, educational packages are provided; gradual re-introductions to activities occur, etc. The authors would like to suggest that the reader pause for a moment here and consider: what do you think would happen if after conducting a thorough risk for myocardial infarction the practitioner then did not proceed to implement a variety of interventions? Or stopped at only preventing the physical means for the person to overstress themselves and administered medications? Yet, as some of the evidence provided in this book has illustrated, sometimes that is precisely what happens with care of the suicidal person. The interventions, if any at all are instigated, predominantly feature preventing the physical means to kill oneself and administering medication.

Various recently produced national suicide strategies are replete with recommendations on how to improve and enhance risk assessment (see for example, Canadian Association for Suicide Prevention 2004, Department of Health 2001, Scottish Executive 2002, Standing Nursing and Midwifery Advisory Committee 1999). These exhortations are laudable, there is a clear need to enhance the accuracy (and frequency of use) of suicide risk assessment, but on its own, this will not be enough. Furthermore, closer inspection of these documents indicates that some recommend that practitioners should use evidence-based interventions to prevent suicide. Again, this seems like a perfectly laudable recommendation, but unfortunately, as a number of authors have pointed out previously (see for example, Maris et al 2000), there is currently a distinct lack of evidence-based interventions for working with suicidal people (though the existence of a limited literature should be noted). What is more concerning to the authors of this book is the continued emphasis on more and more risk assessment with very little reference to what practitioners can or might do once they have undertaken this. The value and necessity of risk assessment notwithstanding, the findings in our study suggest that focusing on risk assessment rather than on caring for (with) suicidal people is an inappropriate focus. The participants in our study were adamant and clear that what they found helpful was not more accurate assessment of risk. The authors wonder if maintaining the status quo of risk as the focus occurs, at least in part, because there is only a limited body of evidence that can guide P/MH nurses on how to work with suicidal people. Perhaps undertaking risk assessments at least gives the P/MH nurse a sense that that are doing something! Whatever the reason(s), P/MH nurses need to spend more time listening to suicidal people, asking where does it hurt, what can I do to help; in essence, re-connecting the person with humanity.

The evidence in this study also suggests that a radical shift in conceptualizations of what constitutes an appropriate time frame for involvement with the person in recovery from a suicidal attempt needs to be achieved. Currently, the emphasis is on assessing risk, managing it through observation (and medication) and moving the person on when an appropriate 'risk score' is achieved. The current study indicates that suicidal people appear to need more long-term support, defined as the maintenance of a relationship based in trust, understanding, co-presence, information sharing and caring. P/MH Nurses must recognize that the suicidal person in recovery is undertaking emotionally demanding work and feels the need for a safety net, even if this is just knowing that s/he can make contact when the going gets tough.

Current models of care for the suicidal person do not appear to account for or allow for this hitherto neglected area. Once the formerly suicidal person is deemed to be at a low enough risk of suicide, it appears that, from the healthcare provider's point of view, the matter of suicide in 'closed', complete or finished. Yet, the evidence in this study (and the alarmingly high rates of suicide soon after discharge) indicates that, for the formerly suicidal person, the matter may not be closed. The impending risk and threat of imminent death is drastically reduced however, there remains much work to be done before the matter can be considered to be 'closed'. Indeed, for some people, the matter may never be closed permanently. The participants in our study explained how they needed to fit together a story that accounts for the way in which the suicidality came into her/his life, its place in the 'here and now' and its trajectory into the future; hard, demanding and long-term work. Participants wanted to and needed to understand the following types of questions:

> 'What meaning does this have for me now? '
> 'How do I weave this experience into the meaning of my life?'
> 'Does this suicidal experience define what I am to be for the remainder of my days?'
> 'What have I learned as a result of this experience?'

Accordingly, additional and perhaps longer term care or interventions need to be provided to the formerly suicidal person in order for them to explore these questions in a non-judgemental, supportive and understanding atmosphere.

To the best of the authors' knowledge, this is an original finding (though we remain open to having this refuted). Further, there are clear links here with the extensive 'meaning making work' that suicide survivors have to engage in (see Chapter 10). Also, we believe that this issue could quite easily be the focus of future study. Just how does a person make sense of the fact that they tried to kill themselves? How does one reconcile this fact with the remainder of one's existence? The preliminary and tentative evidence in our study suggests that there is likely to be more than one process, but there may well be commonalities that transcend individual experiences (hence the need for another GT study). The evidence that can be found in the testimonies of people who have tried to take their own life and did not 'succeed' make for compelling reading (see for example, Teri Wise's excellent book) and indicate that some such individuals have transformed this experience into one that can help others. We return to this point in Chapter 10.

Practice discussion point seven: P/MH nursing care for the suicidal person needs to be based in a 'recovery' and not a 'cure' model

It is naive to think that the person who has made a serious suicide attempt can be 'cured' in the sense of being relieved from a physical disease; there is no 'cure' for life. Rather, the person is working through what suicide means in terms of past, present and future life. This process fits more with the idea of 'recovery'. In order to make this conceptual link more explicit, it is necessary to include a brief examination of the notion of recovery in (or from) mental health problems (though we do acknowledge that suicide is not a mental health problem *per se*).

The notion of recovery in mental health, as Barker and Buchanan (2005) so aptly point out, has become something of the latest fad, 'buzzword' or fashionable term. Within their fine scholarly work the argument is made that recovery may have very different meanings for mental health service users to those held by mainstream psychiatric workers. Recovery, at least in part, is concerned with re-capturing what once was lost; recovery is concerned with revival and/or retrieval. According to Barker and Buchanan (2005) recovery would be better expressed as reclamation. Other synonyms for recovery include: healing, improvement, resurgence, renewal and revitalization.

In the biographical account of Nobel Prize winner John Nash's life (Nasar 1998) including his 'recovery' from serious mental health problems (he was given the diagnosis of schizophrenia), Nash himself, on accepting his prize did not entirely accept the plaudits that he had 'recovered'. Nash made the comments that had he 'only' returned to his pre-diagnosis level of intellectual functioning, this in his view did not constitute recovery; recovery would be epitomized by surpassing this earlier level of intellectual functioning.

Clearly, recovery is a process; it is not a singular event or something that occurs spontaneously 'overnight'. Recovery, especially in the context of mental health problems, appears to be a process that occurs over a number of years. While the authors of this book wish to eschew limiting the duration of recovery according to some pre-determined and forced boundaries, it seems likely that recovery is not a hasty process. Also, recovery need not have an 'end point' *per se*, it can refer to a transformation of the self; the unearthing or discovery of new possibilities. In other words, recovery can be, as Nash argued, an opportunity to go beyond one's former self. Further, as with the previous discussion point, one might speculate that as recovery is another 'human' psychosocial process, it seems likely that there could be commonalities across individual accounts and experiences.

Nevertheless, whether recovery is concerned with reaching a new, higher level of functioning or merely regaining some functioning; whether one's process of recovery is swift or less so, there are clear links here between the apparent processes of recovery and re-connecting the person with humanity. In essence, the suicidal person can be seen to be recovering his/her former functioning, former pre-suicide life; former pre-suicide beliefs, and former emotional wellbeing. There may be additional merit in this conceptualization if indeed the arguments posited about the experiential value of recovery are accurate; namely, that the process of recovery (the process of re-connecting with humanity) can bring about growth beyond the pre-suicidal existential state. These propositions though should be regarded as that – theoretical, and as yet, untested propositions that require additional evidence before they are entered into the substantive knowledge base of suicidology.

Chapter 9

The Bigger Picture – Future Research and Contemporary Mental Healthcare Policy Implications

'Goal 1: Develop, implement and sustain community based suicide prevention programs, respecting diversity and culture, locally, regionally and provincially/territorially. 1.6 The development of training and technical centres to build capacity for provinces, territories, regions and communities to implement and evaluate suicide prevention programs.'
Canadian Association for Suicide Prevention 2004, p 11

'Goal 3: increase training for recognition of risk factors, warning signs and at risk behaviours and for provision of effective interventions, targeting key gatekeepers, volunteers and professionals'.
Canadian Association for Suicide Prevention 2004, p 12

CHAPTER CONTENTS

INTRODUCTION

Having discussed the robustness of the emerging theory and the practice implications arising out of the findings, in this chapter the authors follow Glaser and Strauss' (1967) edict that a researcher should move from the substantive to the formal level. Expanding the consideration of the implications is also appropriate practice for researchers *per se*. The authors also subscribe to an oft stated axiomatic view, namely, that good research should create more questions than it answers. Therefore, this chapter firstly focuses on a number of research questions that arise from our findings. Following this, and bearing in mind the goals/objectives of the Canadian Association for Suicide Prevention (2004) blueprint cited at the start of this chapter, and perhaps moving to the most formal level of discussion, the authors highlight and address a number of policy implications that arise out of our findings.

RESEARCH IMPLICATIONS

The authors have identified five potential studies that would be the logical next steps to take following on the heels of this completed study. In no way do we regard this list as exhaustive (and we hope others will add to it), but we regard these as five subsequent questions that do need to be asked. These are listed in Box 9.1 and then explained in more detail.

Research discussion point one: there is a need for an investigation to determine the current extent of formal education and training for the care of the suicidal person

Despite the fact that suicide continues to be regarded as a major health issue within many countries, including Canada and the United Kingdom, and that certain subgroups (e.g. people with mental health problems, aboriginal Canadians), continue to present with significantly higher risk than the general population, the opportunities for P/MH nurses to receive education/training

---

Box 9.1 Research implications

1. There is a need for an investigation to determine the current extent of formal education and training for the care of the suicidal person.
2. There is a need for an investigation to establish the degree of confidence and competence that clinical staff possess when they are nursing suicidal people.
3. There is a need for an 'action research' evaluation study that examines the skills, attitudes and knowledge base of P/MJ nurses pre and post formal training for care of the suicidal person.
4. Replication(s) of the study described in this book need to occur in a number of additional sites /countries.
5. There is a need for a longitudinal comparison study, between an independent variable group (e.g. suicidal people P/MH nurses who have undergone additional formal training) compared with standard practice group (e.g. P/MH nurses who would focus on the use of observations and medication as the means to 'care for' suicidal people).

in how to care for the suicidal person appear to be scarce. Precise numbers of how many P/MH nurses, past and present, have received formal training/education are currently not available. The apparent remedy for this would be to undertake some form of large-scale national survey. This could (should) be carried out in numerous countries. However, previously in this book we have included evidence that shows how often the people (or discipline) who provide 'care' or 'help' for suicidal people are not registered P/MH nurses (see Chapters 2 and 8). Accordingly, determining the extent of training/education for those who provide care for suicidal people cannot be exclusive or restricted to permanent, qualified clinical staff. Those other disciplinary groups need to be surveyed, too, and the extent of their training/education determined. Accordingly, the national survey would need to determine:

(A) How many clinical staff, be they permanent, part-time, casual, qualified or unqualified, have undertaken care for a suicidal client?
(B) How many of those clinical staff, have received formal pre or post registration training/education in how to care for the suicidal person?
(C) When (if) this training/education occurred?
(D) What was the nature and composition of the training/education?

This survey information could provide important 'baseline' data and provide an empirical, rather than anecdotal, indication of the extent of the problem.

Research discussion point two: there is a need for an investigation to establish the degree of confidence and competence that clinical staff feel/possess when they are nursing suicidal people

In addition to determining the extent of formal education/training provided to P/MH nurses to enable them to work with suicidal people, efforts should also be made to determine how equipped nurses feel when they have to provide care for the suicidal person. Moreover, it would be useful to investigate why some P/MH nurses feel more confident in providing such care than others. The complexity of caring for people who are at risk of suicide is well established. The findings in this study support that already well established position that suicidal people need highly specific, and sophisticated, forms of care, particularly if the P/MH nurse attempts to do more than keep the suicidal person physically safe. Providing such complex and emotionally demanding care makes huge demands on the personal resources of the P/MH nurse. The resultant stress associated with providing such care would be further exacerbated in situations where the P/MH nurse feels that he/she is ill equipped to give this care. Yet, maybe this is something of an assumption on the part of the authors; maybe the degree of confidence has little or no effect on the care provided. However, clearly more empirical evidence is needed to either refute or support the purported and intuitively logical relationship between the P/MH nurse's confidence and the subsequent care offered to the suicidal person.

The relationship between competence and care provided to suicidal people appears to have spontaneous validity. It is difficult to imagine a situation where an increased incompetence in P/MH nurses consistently produces higher quality of care for suicidal people. Nevertheless, more accurate data relating to P/MH nurses' degree of competence would be useful. Particularly if this is investigated more thoroughly around the ideas of what leads them to feel competent and how do they judge that they are?

Research discussion point three: there is a need for an 'action research' evaluation study that examines the skills, attitudes and knowledge base of P/MH nurses pre- and post-formal training for care of the suicidal person

If one accepts that the findings of this study have credibility and utility, and the arguments the authors have made in the 'Practice Discussion Points', then there is a clear need to provide additional and evidence-based education/training for P/MH nurses who wish to care for suicidal people. If this education/training were to occur with no efforts to monitor and evaluate the outcomes, then this would appear to be an intervention with limited value. What appears to be indicated here is an 'Action Research' design for a study that would evaluate the effectiveness of the education/training. Such 'Action Research' designs have already been used with much success to address the problem of high suicide rates in certain populations, such as the study focusing on primary care physicians in Gotland, Sweden (see for example, Rutz et al 1989, 1992a, b).

In these papers it is reported that during the years 1983/5, the Swedish Committee for the Prevention and Treatment of Depression (PTD) organized a postgraduate training programme on the diagnosis and treatment to all the general practitioners on Gotland, Sweden. This analogously formed the 'intervention' aspect of this 'action research'. In keeping with an action research design, the effects of the intervention were then measured over time. As a result, in the years following the postgraduate training programme, the frequency of suicide and inpatient care for depression were measured and these were found to have decreased significantly. The results of the Gotland study produced convincing evidence that early recognition and adequate treatment of depression is one effective method of suicide prevention (Rutz et al 1989, 1992a, b). Thus, it can be seen that action research designs have already been used within suicidology research, that training/education interventions can be provided and systematically evaluated and that these evaluations provide empirical evidence to suggest that improved training/education can indeed reduce the suicide rate.

Research discussion point four: replication(s) of the study described in this report need to occur in a number of additional sites/countries

It was not the intent of this study to produce nomothetic generalizations. It was, however, one of the intentions to produce idiographic findings (for the necessity of both forms of knowledge in understanding suicide, the reader is referred to Leenaars 2004 and Maris et al 2000). To rephrase, the authors were concerned with finding contextually based 'truths', or 'essences' that are understood in terms of the particulars of various cases. As we stated earlier in the book (Chapter 3) this had never been done before; a substantive theory of how UK P/MH nurses provide meaningful caring responses to suicidal people did not exist.

Nevertheless, as we also pointed out in Chapter 3, we acknowledge and embrace Glaser's (1978, 1998) and Glaser and Strauss' (1967) methodological maxim that a modified grounded theory initially produces substantive level theory. It produces what some would term 'local theory', as it brings together and systematizes isolated, individual theory. (Glaser refers to it as an aggregate of local understandings.) As a result, there would be a robust methodological argument and epistemological utility in broadening the scope of the theory by repeating the study in different geographical areas within the UK. It should be noted though that this study would not start 'a-new' with an a-theoretical position, but would be in effect a continuation of the constant comparison method but accessing a different sample.

Similarly, it should be noted that the UK is by no means the only country with a significant suicide problem. For example, in reviewing the largest collection of suicide-related literature in Canada held at the Suicide Information and education Centre (SIEC), not a single Canadian study was discovered which referred to an evidence-based underpinning for providing P/MH nursing care to suicidal patients. Consequently, it can be seen that there is a similar need to undertake the same study as we describe in this report in order to develop a theory for Canadian psychiatric nurses who provide care for suicidal inpatients; including the disproportionately high number of First Nations peoples who are admitted to formal psychiatric care centres.

Research discussion point five: longitudinal comparison of levels of risk between independent variable group (e.g. nurses who have undergone additional formal training) compared with standard practice group (e.g. nurses who would focus on the use of observations and medication as the means to 'care for' suicidal people) are needed

The final logical research question arising from this study would be a study that compares the contemporary standard 'care' of the suicidal person and the proposed model highlighted in this study, on the suicide risk that clients present. Risk assessment, rightly or wrongly, continues to form a major component of care of the suicidal person. Accepting the well documented limitations of risk assessment, there may still be utility in undertaking a study that would show which of the two approaches to caring for the suicidal person reduces the person's suicide risk the most.

This study would have particular value if the suicide risk were gauged over a long period of time. Traditionally, assessment of risk would not continue in earnest once the (former) suicidal person has been discharged. Yet, the evidence in this study indicated a need for a longer-term involvement from the formal psychiatric services. This was the time needed for the person to find the meaning in his/her suicide episode; the time needed to weave this new experience (the suicide episode) into the existing meanings of his/her life. Consequently, if it can be shown that this longer-term involvement of the formal psychiatric services further reduces a person's suicide risk, then the additional implications for practice are clear, particularly, given the significant number of completed suicides that occur in the short time period immediately following discharge.

POLICY IMPLICATIONS

The logical extension of many of the Practice Discussion points outlined earlier would be to formalize these practices into policy. Accordingly, matters such as P/MH nurses moving away from risk-focused work to care-focused work, embracing a radical shift in conceptualizations of an appropriate time frame for care of the suicidal person, moving away from medication-based work to interpersonal care-based work and adopting a recovery and not a 'cure' model, all have potential policy level implications. Furthermore, the need for additional education/training in providing care for the suicidal person has been outlined previously in this book, and accordingly, the resulting policy position would be 'more education/training is needed'. Thus there would be little merit in repeating these implications in this section. Therefore, the authors will focus on four particular related policy implications. These are listed in Box 9.2 and then explained in more detail.

Box 9.2 Research implications

1. 'Treatment' and 'management' of the suicidal person should be driven by the care of the person and not just risk assessment; this may necessitate a wide scale, re-visiting and revision of fundamental conceptualizations of mental health care and mental health care policy.
2. Suicidal people should be cared for by P/MH nurses who have had appropriate training not by casual staff and students with little or no experience.
3. Close observation should be replaced with clinical engagement as a matter of urgency.
4. Clinical supervision for P/MH nurses caring for the suicidal person.

Policy discussion point one: 'treatment' and 'management' of the suicidal person should be driven by the care of the person and not just risk assessment; this may necessitate a wide scale, re-visiting and revision of fundamental conceptualizations of mental healthcare and mental healthcare policy

The authors have previously alluded to this point (see Chapter 8) therefore we do not intend to unnecessarily repeat ourselves here. However, it is worth re-stating that there is a clear need to expand (or change) our current emphasis from one of (only) assessing and managing risk to one of actually providing meaningful caring responses to suicidal people. Let us reiterate here, the authors wholeheartedly embrace the need for comprehensive risk assessment, but that is just the beginning of care for the suicidal person. Accordingly, if there is going to be a fundamental shift in our conceptualizations of what constitutes appropriate care for the suicidal person, then it needs to be underpinned, if not actually driven by, mental healthcare policy. This may not be an easy task to accomplish given that the discernable trend in mental healthcare policy over recent years has been towards more coercion and control (and risk management is clearly bound up with such policy). If there is going to be any change/challenge to this policy, then it is necessary to examine the issue in more detail.

Mental health and mental healthcare policy: a contested area

Rogers and Pilgrim (2001) have rightly drawn attention to the fact that mental health remains a highly contested area. There is little (or no) widespread agreement concerning the nomenclature, let alone the causes and aetiology of mental health problems (see Barker 1997, Dawson 1997, Gournay 1996, Keen 1999, Pilgrim & Rogers 1999). Not surprisingly, a parallel – and linked – debate continues over what the appropriate response(s) should be to people affected by mental health problems (Hannigan & Cutcliffe 2002, p 478). These authors continue:

> 'Frameworks for understanding 'mental illness' that emphasise physical causes tend, logically, to emphasise the importance of physical treatments, such as psychotropic medication. Alternatively, frameworks that emphasise the importance of environmental, social or interpersonal factors in the causation of mental illness tend to emphasise environmental, social and interpersonal interventions.'

There appears to be little disagreement that the way one conceptualizes mental health and mental health problems (for some, mental illness – though this in and of itself is a construct; a certain view), will ultimately be highly important and influential in determining mental healthcare policy, and what type(s) of service people receive when they encounter formal mental healthcare. Moreover, Hannigan and Cutcliffe (2002, p 478) argue that such conceptualizations have a much wider implication:

> 'However, these ideas are also important at another, more macro, level. In particular, ideas about mental health and illness are important in influencing the overarching political and legal frameworks within which services are provided ... the trend in the UK is towards a more controlling and coercive mental health policy. This, we suggest, is a reflection of the idea that mental illness is something that needs to be 'managed' and controlled.'

Interestingly, Heffern and Austin (1999) suggest that the shift towards a more coercive policy is a 'global' one, and evidence certainly exists that indicates the same trend in Canada.

Current mental healthcare policy and its emphasis on masculine approaches to care and managing risk

Even a cursory examination of mental healthcare policy will demonstrate that the dominant way of thinking about mental health and illness is the 'medical' or 'disease' model; coupled with the management and treatment of these 'disorders' (Hannigan & Cutcliffe 2002). Further such policies inevitably focus on 'masculine' approaches to care and we have previously pointed out how this is echoed in the care of the suicidal person policy literature. As a result, the problem of 'suicide' is seen to reside in individuals who thus need to be managed and this inevitably means managing the risk. Further, the 'solution' to the person's suicidality is seen to reside in the hands of the psychiatrist – not necessarily the person themselves.

Recent mental health policy documents continue to emphasize risk and the management of risk. The Department of Health White Paper Reforming the Mental Health Act (Secretary of State for Health and Home Secretary 2000), for example, acknowledge that the vast majority of people with mental illness pose no threat to other people; nevertheless, the document qualifies this statement with the additional remark that Government has a duty to protect individual patients and the public if a person poses a serious risk to themselves or to others (Hannigan & Cutcliffe, 2002). According to Rogers and Pilgrim (2001) this reflects a worldwide trend towards the 'medicalisation' of mental health problems, and the greater concern with managing risk – often through increased use of compulsion (hence the over zealous use of observations). Hannigan and Cutcliffe (2002, p 479) concur:

> 'Despite acknowledgement that the vast majority of those who suffer from mental illness pose no threat to other people, and in many cases are amongst the most vulnerable in society, the clear emphasis in the current UK White Paper is on managing the risk that mentally ill individuals pose to society.'

It seems plausible too that mental health policy is heavily influenced by at least two other phenomena:

1. The mass media (mis)representations of mental health service users, the resultant increase in stigma, ostracism, harassment and victimization and the corresponding public 'outcry' that people with mental health problems need to be better 'managed' (Cutcliffe & Hannigan 2001).
2. The rising fear of litigation and hence the corresponding rise in risk management. Interestingly, Bender (Canadian Psychiatric Association 2004, p 26) notes in *Psychiatric News* that psychiatrists are now being advised on ways to avoid litigation arising from the excessive use of risk prevention interventions (e.g. seclusion rooms and restraint). It seems, not without a sense of irony, that risk management has become in and of itself – a risky and litigious matter! More encouragingly the Joint Commission on Accreditation of Healthcare Organizations has encouraged psychiatric healthcare staff to attempt to create psychological advanced directives. Formal agreements produced with clients to identify various coping strategies and options for care of the client if he/she begins to lose control. So while the mental health care policy literature continues to focus on risk management and defensive practices, at the clinical level some practitioners are attempting to work with the people who use mental health care facilities. In addition to this practice level change, there is a clear need for P/MH nurses and others involved in the formal care of suicidal people to lobby political groups and organizations, under the auspices of the P/MH nurses' macro level of care responsibility, and encourage the suicide policy literature to reflect a less defensive, less risk management oriented position.

Policy discussion point two: suicidal people should be cared for by P/MH nurses who have had appropriate training, not by casual staff and students with little or no experience

The need for well educated and skillful practitioners was highlighted in the findings in this study. The participants were very clear that they drew comfort and hope from the fact that they were cared for by experienced, knowledgeable practitioners. The participants had faith in their P/MH nurse because they had seen 'this type of thing before'. One could be forgiven for thinking that advocating appropriately trained practitioners to provide care for suicidal people is a redundant point; after all, why would anyone advocate for anything else? However, if this is a redundant argument then it makes the current situation *apropos* care of the suicidal person even more difficult to understand. As a result maybe it is necessary to re-state the need for suicidal people to be cared for by highly educated and skilled practitioners. Yet, it would be remiss of the authors to make such recommendations without giving due attention to workforce planning issue and more specifically, the international shortage of P/MH nurses.

Extensive shortages of P/MH nurses across the UK have led to a reliance on 'bank' or agency staff; casual rather than permanent staff. For example, in a recent study by Gournay et al (1998), it was found that bank nurses provided between 23.6 and 36.3% of the staff complement, and the authors quite rightly went on to condemn this practice as unacceptable. While such figures vary in different sites across the UK, this pattern is by no means exclusive to London (Dodds & Bowles 2001). More alarming, it is not isolated to the UK. Figures from Canada indicate that the number of Registered Psychiatric Nurses (RPNs) is steadily decreasing; more worryingly, the average age of RPNs is dangerously close to the mandatory retirement age and it is increasing. If the current trends were to continue over the next decade, it would mean that approximately half the RPN workforce in Canada would disappear. Using the situation in British Columbia to illustrate this point, even producing new RPNs at maximum capacity, the current programmes would not be able replace these retirements, let alone increase the number of RPNs.

Perhaps this situation goes someway to explaining why some key aspects of P/MH nursing practice are now carried out by sitters, security guards and CCTV? Perhaps this explains at least in part, why some organizations are comfortable with focusing on defensive practice as when care of the suicidal person is reduced down to nothing more than a disengaged gaze, then why not replace P/MH nurses with sitters, security guards and CCTVs? The clear evidence of the ineffectiveness of this situation though is difficult to ignore. Defensive practices carried out by people who, through no fault of their own, lack the skills, educational background and training to provide meaningful caring responses to suicidal people is simply inadequate, inappropriate and ineffective.

If this situation and argument is extrapolated to its logical (and extreme) conclusion, it suggests or rather reinforces the need not only for more P/MH nurses internationally, but at the same time, P/MH nurses who have the education, clinical skills, training and personal development required to work effectively with suicidal people. At the risk of sounding melodramatic, the current tragic situation of lost lives – lives that may have been saved had they received more effective care – is simply unacceptable and needs urgent remedial attention.

A possible educational model?

The authors have stated previously in this book that our belief is that the best that can be achieved in pre-registration (basic entry level P/MH nursing preparation) would be an introduction to caring for suicidal people. Further, though clinical mentoring, preceptorship and working in combination with experienced, senior clinicians, student P/MH nurses ought to be able to grasp the basics. The authors firmly believe that additional post-graduate (post-basic) education and training in care of the suicidal person is required. The authors are aware that current post-basic education in this area almost inevitably involves very short 'in-service' training; indeed we have seen training starting from as a little as one half of one day. Further, almost inevitably, the content of such courses focuses on risk, identifying risk factors, and managing risk.

The authors are of the view that much more sophisticated education and post-basic training is needed. At the very least, in order to provide effective, meaningful caring responses to suicidal people, the authors believe a course should contain the following (minimum) elements:

- Self-awareness training – specifically dealing with one's own mortality
- Cognitive re-framing techniques and skills
- Experiential work around being comfortable with stillness
- Monitoring one's self – particularly one's own level of hope
- Experiential work around hearing about death, dying and suicide
- Techniques and qualities associated with inspiring hope
- Presencing
- Listening (without prejudice or discomfort)
- The use of gentle, implicit challenges
- Clinical supervision
- Creating a calming, peaceful external (physical) environment
- Experiential work on becoming comfortable with not having erudite answers
- Interventions and attitudes to build trust
- Interventions geared to explore and facilitate understanding of the meanings attached to the suicidal act (e.g. catalytic interventions (Heron 1990), empathic building, selective reflection).

Policy discussion point three: close observations should be abandoned as a matter of urgency

The authors have already provided substantial evidence that highlights the problems with observations as an approach for 'caring' for suicidal people, therefore, we do not wish to repeat ourselves unnecessarily. Nevertheless, as with Policy Discussion Point One in this chapter, if there is going to be a wide-scale practice-level shift in our conceptualizations of care for suicidal people, then it needs to be underpinned (driven by?) corresponding shifts in the policy literature. Accordingly, the authors recommend an urgent shift in the suicide policy literature; one that replaces observations (and other forms of defensive practice) with more therapeutic, restorative, and recovery focused models such as the theory described in the book.

Sadly, the contemporary P/MH nursing literature is clear in highlighting that all too often, what suicidal people receive in the way of P/MH 'nursing care' is indeed, second rate, ineffective and impersonal. We leave the last words on the matter, fittingly, to the founder of Suicidology as a discrete field of study Ed Shneidman who states:

> 'When dealing with a highly suicidal person, it is simply not effective to address the lethality directly. We can address thoughts about suicide by working with this person and asking why mental turmoil is leading to feelings of lethality'.

Shneidman, 1997, p 25

> 'To understand suicide we must understand suffering and psychological pain and various thresholds for enduring it; to treat suicidal people (and prevent suicide) we must address and then soften and reduce the psychache that drives it'.

Shneidman, 1997, p 29

Policy discussion point four: regular clinical supervision must be provided to nurses caring for the suicidal person

There has long been a consensus that caring for suicidal people, especially if one actively engages with the person rather than observing from a distance, makes huge demands on the well-being of the carer. In addition to these demands, providing such care also makes significant emotional demands on the P/MH nurse, and can have a negative emotional impact on them (see for example, Barker & Cutcliffe 1999, Cutcliffe & Barker 2000, Duffy 1995, Hamel-Bissel 1985, Jobes et al 2000). Further, there appears to be a positive correlation between the level of client/clinician interpersonal engagement (and associated emotional investment) and the extent of emotional load experienced by the clinician. To paraphrase, the more the P/MH nurse gives to the relationship, the greater the demands this makes upon him/her. Even when there is a successful outcome, there is a great deal of stress experienced. Moreover, despite the best efforts of these clinicians, as stated above, some of the suicidal people under care will go on to complete suicide, either during their formal care episode or within the first year after discharge. Such is the incidence that Jobes et al (2000) found that approximately one half of psychiatrists and one quarter of psychologists will lose at least one person to suicide during the course of their careers. Interestingly, despite their high level of contact with suicidal people, the authors could find no such data pertaining to P/MH nurses. In addition to the stress of caring for suicidal people, the stress of losing a suicidal person is understandably worse given the sense of 'failure' that often occurs in such situations. Jobes et al (2000) provide a useful summary of the effects that have been reported in clinicians who have lost a suicidal client, with perhaps the most significant being that the clinician themselves becomes at risk of suicide.

Clearly, the emotional impact or labour of caring for suicidal people, the sophisticated and complex forms of care, and the unique challenges that such people present, and the unfortunate but distinct possibility that a suicidal person may take their own life, necessitates the need for regular clinical supervision (Cutcliffe et al 2001, Stevenson 2005). This would provide the opportunity for the nurses to receive appropriate, regular and restorative support necessary to enable them to continue working with such people. Such structured reflection not only assists the unique challenges to be met but, additionally, it offers the P/MH nurse an opportunity to learn and develop the knowledge, skills and attitudes needed to care for such individuals.

Certain critical incidents within the realm of providing care for the suicidal person may even indicate the need for formal debriefing sessions and further additional forms of support. However, such clinical supervision and formal support mechanisms are not, and have not always been in place. Indeed, the absence of formal support systems is likely to exacerbate the situation where clinical staff have high stress levels, and these levels of stress preclude them from further therapeutic engagement with suicidal clients. Thus, the authors would argue that engaging with suicidal clients reiterates and reinforces the need for nurses involved in such care practices to receive appropriate clinical supervision.

Chapter 10

Whose Life is it Anyway? Ethical Issues in Caring for the Suicidal Person

'Whatever the truth is, we need to be prepared to go where it takes us.'
Maris et al 2000

CHAPTER CONTENTS

INTRODUCTION

There can be few ethical issues that prompt more passionate and polarized debate than those matters pertaining to end-of-life decisions. While on initial consideration, the subject of suicide may appear to be spared the vagaries of such interrogation however, on closer inspection, it can be seen that it is replete with hitherto unresolved ethical dilemmas. As a result, it would be remiss of the authors if we were to write a book that is concerned with care of the suicidal person, without giving due consideration and attention to (some of) the associated ethical issues.

We believe that ethical issues are important topics for consideration for those directly or indirectly involved in the care of the suicidal person; indeed we would regard this position as axiomatic. We will not belabour the obvious connection between the individual practitioner's own ethical and philosophical stance on suicide and the resultant 'care' the suicidal person receives. Yet, it is similarly 'true' that often practitioners may not have given full consideration to their own ethical view, and consequently, may inadvertently be ignorant of the influences on their interactions with and care of suicidal people. Even assuming that practitioners have indeed engaged in self-refection and consideration of their ethical views, it needs to be acknowledged that there is great merit and utility in re-visiting these. This is particularly the case because, as we will demonstrate in this chapter, the ethical issues and their associated discourses pertaining to suicide (and care of the suicidal person) are iterative and dynamic. Moreover, there is additional merit in examining literature emanating from related disciplines since, as Davidson (2003, p 108) so eloquently captures, 'approaching the understanding of suicide exclusively from within one's own discipline is like looking close up at dots in a pointillist canvas'. Not only does this indicate the need for frequent re-examination of the issues and one's own stance/view, but at the same time, the arguments we construct and the positions we outline in this chapter should not be regarded as an 'endpoint' in and of themselves. They represent some current contemporary views; views which might change in the light of future evidence, case law decisions and subsequent ethical discussions. Accordingly, this chapter summarizes and offers up for discussion a number of principal questions which should inform the subsequent ethical discourse around the matter of suicide. These questions are:

- Whose life is it anyway?
- Is suicide ever a rational thing to do?
- Is there such a phenomenon as a rational or appropriate suicide?
- What role, if any, should healthcare practitioners play in assisted suicide?

To help with this end, case law and existing examples from clinical practice will be drawn upon in order to better inform the discussion in the hope that this can contribute to more fully informed ethical standpoints and give rise to more fully informed practice.

It is important to point out that this chapter may well have an 'exploratory sense' to it; it perhaps poses more questions than it answers; the authors make no apologies for that. We recognize and embrace the fact that questions are the beginning of wisdom; that questions ultimately lead to enlightenment. Although, it is also worthy of note that depending on one's moral and/or theological stance, asking and considering these questions may cause a degree of discomfort. Discussing matters of death can often produce strong/powerful emotional responses; this is perhaps even more the case when discussing matters related to suicide. Nevertheless, the authors firmly believe that it is only in being willing to explore these issues that our understanding grows and perhaps, our discomfort diminishes. Together with some of his colleagues, the eminent suicidologist and former president of the American Association of Suicidology, Professor Ron Maris makes this point most clearly when he states:

> *'Whatever the truth is, we need to be prepared to go where it takes us.'*
>
> Maris et al 2000

Therefore, the chapter begins with an overview of the three principal ethical perspectives germane to suicide research, as proffered by Mishara and Weisstub (2005). Following this, the first question is considered, including consideration of the philosophical perspectives *vis a vis* self and body ownership. This section also makes reference to direct and indirect harming of our bodies and the corresponding incongruence and inconsistency in the associated ethical discourses. The idea of the temporary ownership of another's body within the context of suicide is then discussed.

The second question is then addressed and highlights some of the historical and contemporary influences on this debate. The important, if not seminal contribution of Speijer and Diekstra is included and this section closes with an examination of the existing case law. In addressing the third question, we look at the relationship between mental health problems and psychiatric diagnosis and suicide, and cast doubt on the automatic assumption that anyone who makes an attempt on his/her life must *ipso facto* have a mental health problem (or disorder) and resultant psychiatric diagnosis. This section closes by examining the immensely influential views of the eminent suicidologist Professor Ron Maris on the possibility of an assisted suicide. The fourth and final question begins by unpicking what is meant by the term, assisted suicide and what this means in terms of action/inaction for the practitioner. Issues around the idea of making the 'right' choice, if indeed there can ever be a single right choice, are considered and this section concludes by referring to Professional Codes of Conduct in the hope that they provide clear and unequivocal guidelines to practitioners who may find themselves facing these dilemmas.

PRINCIPAL ETHICAL PERSPECTIVES

In their recent paper, Mishara and Weisstub (2005) designate three broad categories of the principal ethical perspectives that are evident within the discourse pertaining to suicide research. Given the not insubstantial overlap between 'clinical issues' and research relating to suicide, here we transplant and employ Mishara and Weisstub's principal ethical positions within the domain of engaging in clinical care with suicidal people. Their three broad principal positions are: Moralist, Libertarian and Relativist.

Moralist

Even a limited examination of the literature germane to the formal care of suicidal people would show the influence of 'the moralist position'. Mishara and Weisstub (2005) indicate that such a position contends that suicide is unacceptable. Accordingly, in any and all situations where the suicidal person is being cared for, the overriding moral obligation is to protect life (and prevent suicide). A number of theological and/or philosophical stand points contain this view on suicide and far from being esoteric or irrelevant to contemporary clinical practice; they are very much operational, influential and even energetic. The oft cited notion that it is a sin against God to take one's life (Aquinas 1945) appears to be tied in to the related issue of body ownership. If one accepts the argument that individuals do not own their bodies, that our bodies are, in effect, 'loaned' to us by God, that life is a gift from God (see below), then it follows that it would be regarded as a sin to take one's own life. In Plato's (1992) *Republic,* he argues that society is composed of many individuals, organized into distinct classes, each of whom occupies a role in providing some component part of the common good. In addition, given that we each have a role to play in ensuring the continuation of said society, we each have a responsibility to society; an individual responsibility to maintaining the smooth operation of the whole society. Suicide, in this sense then, is an act not only against oneself but against one's society as well (given that one has an obligation to society and thus to protect one's life), and thus is regarded as unacceptable. Additional arguments against suicide draw upon Immanuel Kant's philosophy and in particular, his central concept of 'moral philosophy', the categorical imperative. According to Kant, an imperative is a proposition that declares a certain kind of action (or inaction) to be necessary. A categorical imperative then designates an absolute, a maxim that exerts its authority in all circumstances, and is both required and justified as an end in itself. Thus, moralist utilizing Kant's reasoning regard suicide, or rather not engaging in the act of suicide, as a categorical imperative; an (in)action that can never be justified as an end in and of itself. The Moralist position on suicide has been historically pervasive and this is perhaps best evidenced in the suicide related laws of many countries. As Mishara and Weisstub (2005) highlight, it is only in relatively recent history that some (not all) countries de-criminalized suicide. It is interesting to note that in the former Soviet Union, 'suicide' was absent from medical and legal discourse as it was espoused by the then Soviet government that such a problem could not exist in Socialist society (Leenaars 2004). Perhaps this represents a modern day example of Plato's notions of the person's responsibility to society? Also, despite the majority of countries repealing their anti-suicide legislation, in some countries (e.g. India, Lebanon) suicide remains a crime even in today's contemporary society.

Libertarian perspective

Examination of the more recent literature germane to the formal care of suicidal people would show the growing emergence of 'the Libertarian' position. Given the evidence of the dates of the changing legislation relating to suicide, one could be forgiven for concluding that the emergence of the Libertarian perspective was tied in to a growing 'movement' towards increasing individual freedom of choice, personal emancipation and greater individual liberty. Consider, for example, the creation of the original Society for Individual Liberty, the first grassroots libertarian organization was formed in Pennsylvania, 1969. The emergence of the Civil Rights movement in the early 1960s within the United States, and the creation and subsequent growth of the Women's liberation movement, women in the civil rights movements, and other involvements of women in the 1960s–1970s in the USA and the world. It is maybe no coincidence then that suicide was de-criminalized in the United Kingdom in 1961 and in Canada in 1972. According to Mishara and Weisstub (2005), Libertarian perspectives contain a broad range of views including an individual's hedonistic right to commit suicide (though it is difficult to understand the pleasure gained from such an act); to suicide as a reasonable and calculated act to avoid pain. Further views extend this idea that a person's decision to commit suicide need not be to relieve current suffering but may be a rationale, contemplated decision to die (Prado 1998).

It appears that Hume (1711–1776) was among the first Western philosophers to espouse a person's right to take their own life; in Hume's view, suicide was not a sin against God (which was the prevailing orthodoxy at that time) or indeed a sin against society. Hume's notion of suicide as a person's right can be seen in contemporary discussions on suicide, particularly in the views of Humphrey (1991), Diekstra (1992), and the more controversial, Kevorkian (1991). Wherein these views not only regard the person's right to suicide as sacrosanct, but perhaps advocate a more radical approach wherein suicide is promoted under certain circumstances. Mishara and Weisstub (2005) point out that irrespective of the particular justification(s) and argument(s), within the Libertarian view there is no obligation to prevent suicide.

Relativist perspective

While the two previously outlined ethical perspectives perhaps have a dogmatic and rigid approach within the associated suicide discourse, this is not the case with the Relativist perspective. Mishara and Weisstub (2005) indicate that Relativist ethicists determine the 'rightness or wrongness' of suicide, and thus the corresponding obligation to intervene (or not), based by consideration of the contemporary, situational and cultural variables and the anticipated consequences of action/inaction. It follows that the 'decision' of a clinician who adopts a Relativist perspective, may in one instance support an individual's right to suicide and in another instance, deny an individual's right to suicide. Interestingly, Mishara and Weisstub (2005) draw the analogy of the 'general public' as 'common sense' relativists. Perhaps as a result of their reduced familiarity with bio-medical and social science ethical discourses, the general public tends to ascribe different values and thus different resultant actions to suicide in different circumstances. While there appears to be utility in this analogy, a cautionary caveat should be added here which points out that 'common sense' is not that common! As a result, basing our ultimate decisions *vis a vis* supporting or not supporting a person's right to suicide on the basis of the consensus of the general public may not be the most prudent course of action.

It is worthy of note that different Relativists may reach opposing decisions about a particular suicide 'case' even though they are considering the same situational, contextual and cultural variables. In some cases, ascribing greater credibility to the 'needs' of the family or society over the individual's needs and in others, the individuals' rights (over those of the family or society) are upheld. Mishara and Weisstub (2005) go on to consider the principles of Utilitarian approaches to ethics; they suggest that, in this context, decisions about suicide are made by determining the best interests of society, by means of a cost/benefit analysis of the utility. Again, in such circumstances, the eventual outcome is not 'fixed' or determined *a-priori* according to dogmatic principles but can vary according to maximizing the social utility resulting from the suicide/non-suicide. Mishara and Weisstub (2005) summarize the Relativist perspective by suggesting that irrespective of the particular essence of the Relativist's view, each of these perspectives considers that the obligation to protect life varies upon an analysis of the situation.

WHOSE LIFE IS IT ANYWAY? THE ISSUE OF BODY OWNERSHIP

One central question to the debate about suicide and assisted suicide is that of, who owns our bodies? Whose life is it; to whom does it 'belong'? This preliminary question leads seamlessly to a number of related questions such as, Do our lives belong to ourselves, our family, our community, our physician or even our state? Are our lives are own? Are we free to do with them whatever we see fit?

The arguments and resultant practice around the concepts of suicide and assisted suicide are prefaced by recognizing one's position with regard to body ownership. Now it is important to point out that, within the field of bio-medical ethics, a growing literature is emerging that focuses on issues related to body ownership (see, for example, the following references: Battin et al's (1998) seminal work; Werth's (1999) fine edited volume which should be considered required reading for this subject; the comprehensive text of Ten Have et al 1998). Additionally, the use of the human body and its parts in healthcare is an issue of growing importance in that contemporary medicine more and more 'transforms' the body, and makes use of body parts for diagnostic, therapeutic activities and one can thus argue, changes how we think about the matter of body ownership. The authors recognize that there is a linked debate about ownership of body parts, but it falls outside the scope of this chapter to include a detailed examination of that debate. Nevertheless, it is necessary to provide a brief overview of the different philosophical perspectives on human body ownership and these are summarized in the 1998 text of Ten Have et al.

Philosophical perspectives *vis a vis* self and body ownership

The Libertarian philosophical perspective on human body ownership predicates that bodies and body parts may be used only with the explicit permission of the person whose body it is. Further, given that the Libertarian philosophical perspective maintains the full ownership of the body by the private individual, the 'extreme example' of an individual being free to commercialize his/her body parts, is used to underscore the issue of ownership. In other words, if I truly own my body, then it is mine to do with what I choose. The Personalist philosophical perspective offers a slightly different view wherein it defends the idea that a person's body is part of the integrated subject that is the person; while at the same time it is also part of the material world. An extremely interesting slant on the whole philosophical debate *vis a vis* body ownership is presented within the Hegelian approach; where it is propounded that the concept of property is philosophically inappropriate when discussing the human body and body parts. Also a Utilitarian philosophical perspective is presented and, not surprisingly, this view makes the case that bodies can be owned by others rather than the self; principally because if greater benefits for a greater number ensue from 'using' bodies, then there is an ethical justification in owning bodies.

The contemporary standpoint within the suicidology academe and the corresponding legal position in most Western (developed) countries appears to be that the individual person owns his/her own body. (However, it needs to be recognized that, given the wide variation around the world in the laws pertaining to suicide, and the variation in court rulings regarding related matters such as 'abortion', that it would be inaccurate to posit one, unanimous and unchallenged law regarding body ownership.) Perhaps building on the Lockien view that every man has a property in his own person, Narveson (1986) constructs a cogent argument when purporting that we own ourselves; we are slaves neither to any other individual nor to our family, society or country. More (1997) similarly constructs a compelling argument for the case of 'self-ownership' and states: 'My mind and body are not collective resources. They are me and they are mine.'

If this standpoint is accurate, if the accepted axiom is that people do indeed own their own bodies (and thus have the right to do anything they want with them), then the illuminating comments of Maris et al (2000, p 476) are difficult to refute or ignore when they highlight the potential paradoxical situation, namely: *'it's your life but you cannot do anything you want with it!'*.

Self-ownership then, or to rephrase, ownership of one's body has philosophical, psychological, and political aspects and, as one can see below, these aspects are 'played out' in the debates around suicide and assisted suicide. Some authors (More 1997, for example) predicate that self or body ownership is an empowering and emancipatory concept; as a principle it provides for self mastery of our lives. Such a position echoes that of the Libertarian perspectives described above. Yet, these views of body ownership are by no means unchallenged. More (1997) identifies the following threats:

> *'Attacks on the very conditions of self-ownership come not only from the metaphysical but from the political and moral. In the 20th century, various forms of collectivism—the belief that the group (state, race, tribe, humanity) is primary over the individual – have prepared millions to relinquish their personal freedom and responsibility. Altruism – the belief that self-interest is immoral and that morality primarily and fundamentally involves serving others – has erected high barriers to ethical and psychological self-ownership.'*

Even a cursory glance over historical trends will show that personal body ownership is a relatively new concept. Throughout documented history it has been recorded that humans believed they were 'owned' or belong to a God; their bodies, as was sometimes said, were 'on loan' to them. Leaving aside theological arguments, it is only recently that vast numbers of the global population, for example, women, children, slaves and serfs, could politically assert that they owned their own bodies. In most cases, their bodies were the 'property' of another. Further, it should also be acknowledged, that if we consider the global population, this may still be the state of affairs for significant (the majority) numbers of people. Concomitantly, some cultures and people held the belief that they were 'owned' by their sovereign ruler; be it a King, Queen, Chief etc.; that the state could exert ownership of the individual, particularly at times when the state needed the 'human resource' of the person. Clear examples of such times include those of being at war, and the parallel dynamic of conscription. Interestingly, despite the protestations of the War Resistors International Council (2005) regarding conscription, Conscientious Objection and the related imprisonment of citizens who do resist conscription, it should be noted that even in 2005, there are some Western (developed) countries (e.g. Finland) who continue to engage in these archaic practices. This is despite the demands made by the United Nations Human Rights Committee (UNHRC). While both the WRIC and the UNHRC suggest that human rights are not an issue of internal political debate, but inalienable rights of all members of the human family, this and other related issues of body ownership maybe cast doubt on such assertions. Such musings lead More (1997) to posit the enlightening question: 'If the individual does not own his or her own life, what can they own?'.

For many practitioners who work in these Western (developed) countries, maybe the issue of body ownership remains largely moot until one is faced with one of the following situations:

1. You are responsible for the care of a suicidal person who has the physical ability to make an attempt.
2. You are responsible for the care of a suicidal person who does not have the physical ability to make an attempt. The practitioner is then placed in the unenviable position(s) of maybe needing to assume temporary ownership of another's body (life), or needing to consider a person's request for you to assist him/her with active means to end his/her life. It is perhaps redundant of the authors to state here that such positions require a huge amount of thought, deliberation, consultation and debate, irrespective of the actions one prefers. Further, such considerations do not occur in isolation of, or are not (should not be) ignorant of associated issues, accordingly, there may be merit in broadening our examination of these matters. Accordingly, in considering these associated debates, mental health practitioners (including P/MH nurses) avoid the insularity of their own disciplines; as Davidson (2003, p 108) points out, 'shared territory begins to show new features when orienting; and marks are examined from other disciplines'.

Direct and indirect harming of our bodies and the corresponding ethical discourses: incongruence and inconsistency

If we adopt the position stated above, that a person owns his/her own body to be axiomatic, though even such a position may be simplistic and inaccurate, this position serves as a useful starting point. Consider then a number of activities that we engage in with our bodies and similarly, consider also the corresponding ethical 'outcry' (or absence of the same) that results in response to the behaviours.

There are plenty of examples where activities (which inevitably involve using one's body) can indirectly result in physical harm to one's body. That is to say that the objective or purpose of the activity is not to harm oneself; but there are risks associated with the activity that can result in harm, e.g. any contact sport – ice hockey, rugby, etc. Yet, it is very difficult to imagine anyone being prevented from engaging in such sports on the basis that they might seriously injure their bodies or in rare circumstances – die. In these cases the individual clearly owns his/her body and can subject it to harm without any resulting ethical or moral 'outcry'.

Then there are those examples of activity where the chance of serious physical injury, if not death, exists as a very real potential outcome; particularly as a result of a mistake or error in judgment. Extreme sports are a good example of this, for example, mountaineering, extreme skiing, etc. As a mountaineer and climber, the first author can attest to often being in situations where one slip in performance or error in judgment would have resulted in his death. As within contact sports, the person engaging in extreme sports is free and able to make those decisions without ethical 'outcry', even though the outcome can be, and often is, the person's death.

Furthermore, in both these 'sporting' examples, there are incidents of people who perhaps lack the physical means themselves to engage or participate in the activity independently; in order to participate they require the physical (and sometimes holistic) support of another person. For example, many is the time the first author has witnessed mountain guides assisting people with mountaineering who, arguably, would lack the prowess and ability to climb independently.

Then there are those activities which have been demonstrated empirically to have a statistically significant effect on shortening a person's life and/or increasing the risk of an early death. Such activities include, but are not restricted to, smoking tobacco, abstaining from physical exercise, and eating a high fat/high sugar content diet (Metz 2006; Surg 2006). Despite the well documented pleas of many a cardiovascular physician, an exercise 'guru' or a dietician, there does not appear to be any substantive ethical argument against a person being able to 'treat/abuse' his/her body in these ways. In these circumstances, the body, well and truly, belongs to the person. While one could theoretically smoke oneself to death, or over indulge/abstain from exercise to the point of it becoming life threatening, we doubt that many deaths resulting from these behaviours would be recorded as 'suicides'. Now, clearly the matter of intent is a crucial factor here (Silverman 1997) as is the duration of the behaviour. Still, in these cases, the person clearly owns his/her own body and can 'treat/abuse' it to the point of causing his/her death. Furthermore, anyone who has been involved in providing healthcare for a long time is likely to have encountered people who are physically unable to obtain tobacco or high fat/high sugar foods independently. However, assisting the person in obtaining these goods is unlikely to result in the practitioner being accused of assisting in the person's death.

Temporary ownership of another's body, self-harm, suicide and paternalism

Next, it is worth considering issues of body ownership for those people who habitually engage in self-harming behaviour. For the sake of this debate, the authors are accepting the well established and extant argument that the dynamics of habitual self-harming and suicidal behaviour are NOT the same (see Kinmond and Bent 2000, Krietman 1977, Santa Mina and Gallop 1998). Arguably, the principal difference between habitual self-harming and genuine suicide attempts is that while suicide is a death orientated action (e.g. the intent is to die) this is not the case with self-harming. Wherein self-harm has been defined as, any non-fatal act in which an individual deliberately causes self-injury or ingests a substance in excess of any prescribed or generally recognized therapeutic dose (Krietman 1977). It has been argued that this definition is broad and could be criticized on the grounds of being non-specific. Perhaps this next definition is more concise: 'Self-harm is commonly defined as an individual's intentional damage to a part of his or her body, without a conscious intent to die, although the result might be fatal'.

A thorough examination of the literature in this substantive area will indicate that, certainly historically, many of the definitions constructed for suicide, parasuicide and self-harm, overlap and yet conflict with one another. However, the large majority of more contemporary empirical work distinguishes parasuicide and self-harm from suicide and suicidal ideation. Indeed, it has been pointed out that the confusion surrounding these terms is heightened by the inclusion of 'suicide' in the word parasuicide, since suicide inherently implies a death wish, thus this is misleading. Consequently, as a result of this conceptual confusion and resultant overlap, it might not be surprising that attitudes towards people who make genuine suicide attempts can 'spill over' or can similarly be invoked when considering the population of people who self-harm.

What strikes the authors as interesting about this behaviour and the resultant response of some carers is the common paternalistic overtures; the often disapproving 'stance' and thus implicit message that such people really do not have permission (and thus the matter goes to body ownership) to harm themselves; and again, such attitudes and shift in body ownership are commonplace when one considers the prevalent *modus operandi* and established orthodox for providing 'care' for the suicidal person. Once under the purview or governance of some other authority (e.g. prison warden, psychiatric nurse, psychiatrist) then the ownership of one's body becomes a more 'blurred' matter.

There is a large and substantial body of literature related to this area which indicates that a range of negative responses to self-harming and suicide related behaviours are commonplace (see Anderson et al 2003, Duffy 1995). Comments from Professor Links's recent study of suicidal, substance abusing men presenting to an urban emergency department capture the negative interactions between patients and staff:

One patient indicated: 'but the way some of the nurses go on, it's like they'd be glad to pass you the gun or scalpel to get you out of their hair.'

Another patient spoke about 'My last suicide attempt, when I was here (specific hospital) there was two doctors and one doctor, he was pretty caring, and the other doctor was like cold-hearted, his name should have been ice cube.'

People who engage in self-harm behaviours often cause feelings of frustration and anger in their formal carers as one emergency physician responded: 'I think there are a lot of us, docs, nurses, other health workers, who feel very used and manipulated by this population.'

Drawing on Berne's (1962) theory of transactional analysis, they often usher the interpersonal transaction into that of parent (formal caregiver) to child (self-harmer); and some practitioners will blur the boundaries of body ownership by imposing various types of restriction. Even a cursory examination of the extant literature pertaining to care of the person who self-harms will show frequent references to 'denying access', 'removing means'. Accordingly, the clear though implicit message here is one of:

> 'You do not have ownership of your body; it is not yours to do what you want with it (e.g. self-harm); when you can demonstrate the 'correct' behaviours to the authority, then we can return ownership of your body to you.'

In the above mentioned study, one suicidal man recalled:

'They didn't put handcuffs on me in the beginning – only when I said I wanted to go out (of the ED), that I needed to smoke and could somebody take me outside. No, everybody was busy, blah, blah, blah, so look, I'm going myself. So they called this guy from security who brought me to the bed and put handcuffs on me.'

What is particularly ironic is that, if we compare the seriousness and extent of the damage caused by (a) people who engage in contact sports, and more so, who engage in extreme sports, and people who habitually over-indulge/under-exercise with, (b) people who self-harm, almost inevitably the physical damage occurring in the 'former' category is far more seriousness than that occurring in the cases of people who self-harm. Yet, inversely, the ensuing actions relating to body ownership and corresponding ethical debate are most often more Draconian and paternalistic in the cases of self-harm than it is in the 'sporting' activities. It would be seriously imprudent then to posit a simple causal positive correlation between the potential seriousness and/or extent of bodily harm and the degree of paternalistic removal of an individual's rights to personal body ownership. There is a clear and obvious lack of congruence between the extent and seriousness of damage and the resultant discourse vis a vis body ownership. This incongruity leads then to alternative explanations and questions. One might speculate that the often posited 'relationship' between suicide and self-harming behaviour, particularly given the inappropriate clustering and categorizing of these behaviours as related in intent, only different in severity, has (and is) contributed to the transference of paternalistic responses to suicide to paternalistic responses to self-harming.

Even if we accept the position that a person owns his/her own body to be axiomatic, it is probable that any mental health practitioner who has worked in a clinical setting will have been privy to scenarios where the person's rights to his/her own body are usurped. There are ample examples of ownership of one's body being overtaken by someone else, e.g. a P/MH nurse, a psychiatrist; albeit, overtaken temporarily. Indeed, the 'power' to assume ownership of other people's bodies is enshrined in the mental health law of numerous countries (see for example Gray & O'Reilly 2001 and the Mental Health Act 1983). Furthermore, in the UK and elsewhere throughout the world, the policy and legal frameworks that surround the provision of mental healthcare are becoming increasingly coercive. For example, emerging mental health policy in the UK includes a commitment to the introduction of compulsory treatment in the community (Hannigan & Cutcliffe 2002, O'Brien & Farrell 2005, O'Reilly et al 2000). Thus the potential for the ownership of one's body to be usurped by another (under the auspices of mental health law) is increasing and becoming more commonplace. Also, it needs to be noted that there are ample examples of when assuming the temporary ownership of another person's body resulted in a positive outcome and the thanks/appreciation of the person, e.g. when the basic rights of suicidal people are removed, forced hospitalization, restricted access to means and the person recovers to the extent that they thank the formal mental health carers. This anecdotal evidence notwithstanding, the interesting question then becomes, when (if ever) does one's ownership of one's body become altered to the extent that choices about life/death/suicide are no longer our own? A response to this question resides, at least in part, by considering the next question and this forms the next section of this chapter; can suicide ever be the reasonable thing to do?

Is suicide ever the reasonable thing to do?

The authors stated in the introduction to this chapter that the discourses (and associated resultant positions) pertaining to suicide are not static; this is very well exemplified in the discourses surrounding the question of, 'is suicide ever the reasonable thing to do'. It is interesting that views on this question have changed over the years, yet perhaps the particular contexts and justifications for when suicide is the 'reasonable thing' also appears to have changed. An interrogation of the relevant theoretical and ethical literature in this area suggests that the contemporary arguments that advocate that suicide *can be* the reasonable thing to do (see Werth & Holdwick (2000) for an excellent review). Such a position appears to be bound up with the significant advances in medicine; the connected ability to keep people alive artificially for longer; and not surprisingly the previously documented increase in accepting the personal liberty of each individual. Indeed, according to one of the pioneering 'voices' for upholding a person's right to suicide, Rene Diekstra (1992), as we gain increased control over biological life, as a result of the progress in medical treatment, the elusive ethical issues of the right to die, will be forced upon us. Leenaars (2004, p 399) makes similar remarks when he states: *'More and more often, the question will be posed whether life or death is the humane choice (in the terminally ill)'*.

Such is the profound nature of these debates that they have the potential to change our very definition of what is and what is not considered to be a suicide (Leenaars & Diekstra 1997).

Historical and contemporary influences

How this question is answered is very much determined by one's cultural and philosophical position and, if one examines the literature relating to the history of suicide, by the prevailing orthodoxies of any given moment in time. Minois' (2001) searching and illuminating text indicates a range views on the 'rightness' or 'wrongness' of suicide. According to Minois (2001) in ancient (or 'classical') Greece and Rome, suicide was considered to be acceptable; further, it was even regarded as an act of heroism under certain circumstances. For the ancient Greeks and Romans then, suicide was, at times, the right thing to do. Interestingly, following the rise and not insubstantial influence of Christianity, suicide was unequivocally condemned. Minois (2001) declares that in historical Christian theology, suicide was regarded as 'self-murder' and what's more, an insult to God. Such pervasive views are still very much in evidence today and are far from limited to countries that profess to hold Christian values. Within the European period of history referred to as 'the Renaissance', suicide began to shift from the purview of the ecclesiastical authorities and become, additionally, a philosophical issue. Minois (2001) then points out that the term self-murder (which had hitherto been the accepted phrase) was superseded by the term suicide; this has been the accepted term ever since. However, a contemporary view is that maybe, in some very specific and finite in number cases, suicide can be the reasonable thing to do. Nonetheless, even the contemporary literature is replete with expressed concerns and the consensus view is certainly not shared by all (see Maltsberger 1998, Silverman 2000, Westfield et al 2000).

The sometimes controversial, but always stimulating views of the psychiatrist (and Libertarian) Thomas Szasz (1985, 1990) can readily be located as supporting the notion that suicide *can be* the right thing to do. Szasz (1985, 1990) is adamant that suicide is not an illness, and the absence of a formal diagnosis within the DSM IV manual appears to support Szasz's views. Suicide, for Szasz, is an act of a moral agent; accordingly, the only person responsible is the person him or herself. Again, such views are synchronous with those upholding the individual's absolute right to personal body ownership. Szasz (1985, 1990) continues, because suicide is perceived (by some) as an undesirable act or event, the same people will thus insist on holding someone or something responsible for it. In other words, for those who believe that suicide can be the right thing to do, when suicides occur, there is a need to apportion blame, there is a need to hold some accountable. Moreover, Szasz (1985, 1990) argues that there is neither philosophical nor empirical support for viewing suicide as different, in principal, from other acts (e.g. getting married/divorced, eating filet mignon, or smoking tobacco). Perhaps two of Szasz's (1985, 1990) more controversial positions on suicide are (a) if the suicidal person does not want help and actively rejects it, the psychiatrist's duty ought to be to leave him alone and (b) if suicide is a basic human right (and such views again echo those regarding personal body ownership) then ought anyone attempt to engage in suicide prevention, as that would be preventing someone from upholding one of their basic human rights?

The required conditions: Speijer and Diekstra's seminal contribution

Relatively recently, Speijer and Diekstra (1980) produced a list of 'conditions' which they believed, constituted a legitimate case for when suicide might *NOT* be prevented. That is to say, when a person could make the case that he/she satisfied each of these criteria, then suicide *would be* the right to do.

The conditions were described as follows:

- The choice of ending life by suicide is based on a free-will decision; not made under pressure.
- The person is in unbearable physical or emotional pain with no improvement expected.
- The wish can be identified as an enduring one.
- At the time of decision the person is not mentally disturbed.
- No unnecessary and preventable harm is caused to others by the suicide.
- The helper should be a qualified health professional and an MD if lethal drugs are prescribed.
- The helper should seek professional consultation from colleagues.
- Every step should be fully documented and the documents given to the proper authorities.

While on initial inspection the list may appear to be comprehensive and helpful, a more detailed consideration shows that there are many associated problems; crucially, many of the 'conditions' or more specifically, whether or not the conditions are met, requires a judgment call. At the risk of sounding pedantic, some of the problems include the following:

- Would the pressure of one's own inevitable and pending death constitute a 'pressure' in and of its self?
- While it may well be unlikely, given the technological advances in many spheres of medicine, pain that has no expectation for improvement 'today' – may have a possibility for improvement 'tomorrow'.
- How long does the 'wish' have to be present for it to be considered to be enduring?
- For some (NOT the authors of this book), the desire to take one's own life is enough evidence to warrant a diagnostic label and thus be categorized as mentally disturbed – although it is vital to realize that there is no 'diagnosis' of suicide in the DSM IV.
- According to conservative estimates, each individual case of suicide affects over 150 people. It seems likely then that somewhere in this sample of people, someone will be harmed.
- While we entirely agree with the utility in and sense of consultation, this can equally lead to conflicting views rather than consensus.

Perhaps building on this original and seminal contribution, other authors have similarly questioned this list and produced their own. One of the most signifi-cant contributors to this area, Werth, produced his own list (Werth 1996).

Existing case law

Next we turn to the existing case law in the hope that this provides some addi-tional clarity to our question: can suicide ever be a reasonable thing to do? As with other elements within this broader debate, the existing case law is equiv-ocal, inconsistent, and highly variable according to its point of origin. That being said, there is perhaps a discernable recent trend towards the position that in certain, very specific situations, case law supports the view that suicide *can* be a reasonable thing to do. In Holland, for example, no healthcare professional who carefully observed Speijer and Diekstra's (1980) rules and conduct for assisted suicide has ever been prosecuted or put on trial (according to Leenaars 2004). This is despite the fact that assistance with another's death (also known as assisted suicide) remains punishable by law. Some countries have no legislation on assisted suicide, let alone case law (e.g. China, India). Where as other countries (e.g. United States of America) have conflicting laws depending which state one draws the case law from and which Supreme Court rulings one examines. Consider that, in 1997, the Supreme Court of the USA ruled that there was no constitutional right for physician assisted suicide (Leenaars 2004). However, the matter of assisted suicide was subsequently passed down to each individual state. This has resulted in prosecution for homicide of a physician who participated in several assisted suicides in one state (e.g Jack Kevorkian, Michigan). Whereas in the state of Oregon, their 1998 act states that a physician is permitted to prescribe a lethal medication to a patient who meets certain conditions (Leenaars, 2004); conditions not surprisingly, very similar to Speijer and Diekstra's (1980) rules. A notable difference between the state of Oregon's conditions and Speijer and Diekstra's (1980) and Werth's (1996) rules, is that the state of Oregon stipulates that the person (in need of assisted suicide) must not be suffering from a psychological disorder or depression. Whereas there already exists a documented case of an assisted suicide in Holland for a 'depressed' woman whose son had just died (Leenaars 2004).

In the United Kingdom, there is even less existing case law to draw upon to make informed judgments. The British Medical Association (2005) state that euthanasia is illegal in the United Kingdom, and that UK law also prohibits assisting with suicide. While the 1961 'Suicide Act' decriminalized suicide in England and Wales, assisting a suicide is a crime under that legislation. The Act states that:

> 'A person who aids, abets, counsels or procures the suicide of another, or an attempt by another to commit suicide, shall be liable on conviction on indictment to imprisonment for a term not exceeding fourteen years'
>
> British Medical Association 2005

The British Medical Association (2005) indicate that in recent years various efforts to produce a legal framework for euthanasia or assisted suicide have been undertaken, but none have succeeded in gaining widespread acceptance. An important example of this is the Doctor Assisted Dying Bill (1997). If this bill had been passed, it would have enabled a person suffering distress as a result of terminal illness or incurable physical condition to obtain a doctor's assistance in ending life. More recently, after spirited debate from both sides on the issue of assisted suicide, the proposal by Lord Jaffe was defeated by a 148–100 vote (Reynolds 2006). It is extremely interesting that existing case law in related (e.g. the doctrine of 'double effect', active euthanasia, withdrawing active treatment) cases, 'paints' a somewhat different picture to that of the current UK law. In the (R v Adams [1957] Crim. LR 365) case, a physician was acquitted of murder charges. Then in 1992, the now infamous case of Dr Cox (R v Cox (1992) 12 BMLR 38) indicates that despite administering a lethal dose of potassium chloride to a dying patient (note: at the request of the patient and her family), Dr Cox was convicted though on a lesser charge of 'attempted murder'. However, despite the guilty verdict, Winchester Crown Court imposed a suspended sentence, the General Medical Council let him off with a 'reprimand' and he is still practising medicine in Hampshire. Lastly, in 1993, the Tony Bland (Airedale NHS Trust v Bland [1993] 1 All ER 821) case concerned the request to withdraw artificial nutrition and hydration. The judgement in that case reflected the view that a decision to withdraw or withhold medical treatment when it cannot confer a benefit, including artificial nutrition and hydration, is not unlawful (British Medical Association 2005). One final note, while there is existing, albeit limited case law pertaining to physician assisted suicide, there appears to be no existing case for regarding psychiatric (or any other nurses) engaging in assisted suicide.

In summary of this section, whether or not suicide is ever a reasonable thing to do clearly depends on one's own theological and philosophical views. Further it also depends on where one happens or chooses to practise. What is more, these two broad categories of variables can be in conflict with one another and this point is emphasized by Kopala and Kennedy (1998, p 25) who state:

> 'despite the existence of a statutory scheme and state licensing requirements, emerging constitutional guidelines, public opinion and the nursing profession's standard of care, in the final analysis, a nurse's decision to participate in assisted suicide may rest on the practitioner's own set of moral values and beliefs.'

Is there such a phenomenon as a rational or appropriate suicide?

Perhaps the orthodox position for some on this point has been, and maybe still is, that there can be no such thing as a rational suicide. Maris et al (2000) draw attention to the widely held view in the 'general public' that anyone who wishes to take their own life must be irrational; for many in the general population, the desire to take one's own life is immediately associated with 'madness'. As a result, in this view, rational suicide is an oxymoron. Now it needs to be stated that a wide range of studies have concluded that having certain mental health problems (or diagnoses) has a clear statistical positive correlation with increased risk of suicide (see for example, Barraclough et al 1974, Beautrais et al 1996, Fawcett et al 1987, Harris and Barraclough 1998, Morgan and Priest 1991, Pokorny 1983, Powell et al 2000, Young et al 1994 – to name but a few.) However, there is a parallel body of literature that highlights a number of problems with this literature and thus casts doubt on the view that ALL people who attempt suicide must have a mental health problem.

Suicide, mental health problems and psychiatric diagnosis: an axiomatic relationship?

In no particular order of priority, we highlight the following problems with the immediate and automatic assumption with the literature that purports that all people who attempt suicide must have a psychiatric illness (and diagnosis):

1. Difficulties in defining when some one does (does not) have a mental health problem;

2. Systems of providing psychiatric care that necessitate all people presenting at psychiatric services must receive a psychiatric diagnosis;

3. Methodological limitations –such as biased sampling.

   a) The psychiatrist van Pragg (2004), who is a noted international psychiatrist and a major contributor to issues related to diagnosis and classification of mental health problems highlights the not insignificant problems in differentiating between 'real' or 'clinical' depression and sadness/distress/mourning. David Greenberg makes similar remarks when he points out how the diagnosis of mental illness is far from an exact science. Accordingly, determining when a person does have a mental health problem (for some mental illness) which leads to a clear cut, precise psychiatric diagnosis is problematic, not in the least because no such clearly demarcated boundaries exist (van Pragg 2004). van Pragg (2004) continues, and using 'depression' as an example, he purports that the problem is not so much defining a 'case', as defining the 'non-case', and indicating where distress and worrying end and 'case' depression begins.

   > 'The border then, between sadness/distress and depression is blurred, and psychiatry so far, has failed to study this issue systematically . . . that border, if such a zone exists at all, is phenomenologically defined (original emphasis) and poorly studied. Mourning, for instance, may and often does, produce a mental state undistinguishable from major depression.'
   >
   > van Pragg 2004

   b) Along with many noted suicidologists and scholars, including Motto (1972), Szasz (1990), Battin et al (1998), Werth (1996) and Werth and Holdwick (2003), Professor of Psychiatry at the University of Calgary, Dr Brian Tanney draws attention to the marked under-reporting of suicide and that the vast majority of suicides do not access formal mental healthcare services. Those that do present with a suicidal act or behaviour, given the design and *modus operandum* of psychiatric services, must be given (or receive) a formal psychiatric diagnosis before discharge. This situation is exacerbated in the United States whereby insurance companies will not pay for treatment unless a diagnosis is recorded. Tanney (2000) points out that this requirement will clearly lead to over-estimates of the numbers of people with psychiatric diagnoses who have also engaged in suicidal acts.

   c) Numerous methodological limitations have been recorded with epidemiological studies that attempt to determine the incidence of suicide in populations of people with mental health problems/disorders – including, sampling bias, problems of definition – e.g. when does a suicidal act become a suicidal act?, the exclusion of actively suicidal people from controlled trials (Mishara & Weisstub 2005), and the various conceptualizations of suicide as an individual or societal issue.

Maris on rational suicide

Professor of Psychiatry Ron Maris, former Director of the Centre for the study of suicide, former president of the American Association of

Suicidology and Editor Emeritus of the journal *Suicide and Life Threatening Behavior*, has argued that there CAN be a rational suicide. Maris et al (2000) contend that all suicides are committed by people who are not thinking clearly, depressed, influenced by substance(s), impulsive, stressed and isolated from loved ones. *They continue with the powerful yet illuminating statement that most people who commit suicide are sad, but they are not necessarily clinically depressed* (our emphasis).

In his inaugural address as President of the AAS, Maris offered a compelling argument for the case of rational suicide. Maris argued that under the best of conditions, life is short, periodically painful, fickle, often lonely and anxiety provoking (Maris 1982). All human beings share the following experiences: mortality (finite), sickness, pain, fickle and unpredictable lifecourse, psychological burdens and stress, mental health difficulties (in whatever form these take – anxiety, low moods, etc.) (Maris 1982). More latterly, Maris et al (2000, p 462) stated:

> *'All meaningful things in our lives (love, marriage, good friends, sexual euphoria, money, property, power, achievement, work success, art and music, religion, drugs, travel, play etc.) are relatively ineffective defenses against death – cynically, they are merely postponements, deferrals and distractions.'*

Related arguments have been made several years ago, and more recently. The holocaust survivor and noted psychotherapist, Victor Frankl (1959) has argued that life, almost inevitably, is about suffering. Cutcliffe (2005) endorsed this view and asserted that depression is an essential piece, if not maybe even a necessary component, of the human experience. We can no more deny this existential state of being than we can any other. Furthermore, the pivotal developmental task and immense experiential value of accepting the limitations of life and learning that life can never be perfect, is inextricably bound up with the experience of being depressed. Maltsberger (2004) makes this point most poignantly when he states:

> *'successful adulthood demands that one must passively endure disappointment over and over again. . . . Maturity demands that one must accept passive suffering without flying into rages against life or against one's body'.*

Consequently, perhaps, given the existential truth of our existence, a more critical question that we should ask is: why do more of us NOT commit suicide?

For Maris and others then, the human population shares an existential truth in that life can be harsh, it is likely to involve pain and suffering, and it will always be finite, nevertheless, however, the huge majority of people do 'endure' this existence; do find solutions and ways to cope; do develop non-suicidal solutions for adapting to the human condition (Maris 1982). However, in the light of these existential truisms, it begins to become more understandable why, for the few, the option of death (of suicide) becomes a rational choice. The more enlightened, contemporary view within the suicidology academe then becomes: suicide does NOT necessarily equate with irrationality OR mental illness; though it is abundantly clear that it CAN.

In summary of this section, and as a way to minimize any potential confusion, we need to clarify our position on this issue. The authors are in agreement that there IS a clear link between mental health problems (or mental disorder) and suicide acts, increased suicidality and increased risk. However, it should be acknowledged that:

> 'For the majority of suicidal acts, mental disorders may be a necessary but not sufficient element. The suicidal process (or trajectory of suicide) is not, however, synonymous with mental disorder phenomenology'
>
> Tanney 2000, p 341

Further, when the methodological, epidemiological and theoretical problems associated with the body of literature purporting a direct causal link between mental disorder and suicide acts, it would be imprudent and epistemologically premature to assume that ALL people who engage in suicidal acts must have a mental health problem/illness.

What role, if any, should healthcare practitioners play in assisted suicide?

It feels inherently 'wrong' as a healthcare professional to be advocating for death – albeit, advocating for an individual's right to assisted suicide. After all:

> 'Life does not seek death, death is not the purpose of life'
>
> Maris et al 2000, p 463

The United Kingdom Nurses Midwifery Council (2004) stipulates that it is the duty of the registered nurse to protect and support the individual health of clients. Yet in the same document, nurses are reminded of their duty to respect the individual rights of the person, and respect their human dignity. Interestingly, both of which have been used as arguments *for supporting assisted suicide*, not opposing it. Nevertheless, few credible health care practitioners would dispute that is incumbent upon them to promote health and well-being.

The American Nurses Association (1994) has made more specific statements than the United Kingdom NMC, and went as far as to offer a position statement on assisted suicide. This documented stated categorically that nurses should not participate in assisted suicide as it would be a violation of their professional code and of the ethical traditions of the profession. But it is worth considering what actions would actually constitute assisting in someone's suicide; what does assisted suicide actually mean?

What does assisted suicide actually mean?

Kopala and Kennedy (1998, p 19) have identified three criteria that need to be present for an act to be considered as assisted suicide. These are:

1. The nurse must know the person intends to end his/her life.
2. The nurse must make the means to commit suicide available to the person.
3. The person must then end his/her life.

It strikes the authors that even these three criteria are likely to be subject to a range of interpretations and thus deciding if the criteria have been fulfilled will be problematic. For example, apriori judgements about suicidal intent are notoriously fickle and can be inaccurate. According to various epistemologists, philosophers and theorists, there are a number of different 'ways of knowing'. Accordingly, to which of these do the criteria refer to? The second criterion is even more subject to interpretation; what does making the means available mean? While apparently obvious in some cases (e.g. providing a lethal dose of pharmaceuticals/poison, physically helping a person into a car, closing the windows and turning on the engine), there are less 'obvious' cases where action may still be interpreted as providing the means. For example, providing information on the most effective ways of committing suicide could be providing the means. Give the proliferation of 'suicide information' web sites on the internet, the authors wonder if showing a person how to search the internet, especially if one already knows that the person has a high risk of suicide, might then be considered as providing the means?

Important though perhaps subtle differences do exist between assisted suicide and euthanasia. It could be argued, therefore, that assisted suicide may be less open to potential abuse than euthanasia because the patient's cooperation must be verified by witnesses at various stages which can be separated in time. The 1994 Oregon legislation, for example, permitted doctors to prescribe a lethal dose for competent patients with a life expectancy lower than 6 months. The patient had to make a witnessed written statement plus two separate oral requests with waiting periods of up to 15 days between requests. The patient had to be referred for counselling to a specialist if depression or a psychological disorder were suspected (British Medical Association 1998).

As legislation *vis a vis* suicide has moved away from suicide as an illegal act (in many countries), and into the domain of formal mental health care, the subsequent duty and responsibility has moved onto the healthcare professional. Accordingly, although the nuances of this responsibility varies from country to country (Leenaars 2004), it is now enshrined in professional and legal statutes that mental healthcare practitioners do currently have a duty or responsibility of care to this client group. As a result, practitioners have both a professional duty and a legal responsibility to make (informed) judgements concerning the care of the suicidal person and these decisions inevitably need to take account of the preceding arguments in this chapter; practitioners need to decide whether or not they are going to engage in assisted suicide and such decisions are rarely straightforward.

Making the 'right' choice?

It is accepted by the suicidology academe that decisions about suicide clearly involve the affect; an affect can and does distort judgment (Maris et al 2000). Indeed, it is well documented that people with mental health problems (or some people with mental illness) have, at times, severe limitations in making fully informed decisions. This has led to, over the years, such people being excluded from being able to comment on their own care and treatment; being unable to refuse medication on the grounds of non-compliance; and being unable to decide for themselves as to what is in their own best interest. This dynamic is never more clearly evident than in the case of suicidal people. However, it must be acknowledged that, perhaps of the constricted way in which suicidal people view their world (Shneidman 1997), such people cannot often see their best alternative to suicide; and suicide is usually (though not always) not the BEST alternative to resolve the human condition (Maris et al 2000). As a result Shneidman offers the pithy yet highly meaningful advice in suggesting that you should never kill yourself when you are depressed! Further, such potentially impaired decision making processes are at least part of the reason why those advocating for an individual's right to assisted suicide are abundantly clear in stating the need for comprehensive screening for mental health problems in anyone seeking assisted suicide.

Judging what is (or was) the right thing to do in these cases of suicide, assisted suicide and care of the suicidal person is determined using what the community defines as 'good' and/or appropriate standards of care and according to Leenaars (2004), the community standard of suicidologists refers to what reasonable similarly qualified practitioners would have done. In terms of nursing decisions related to care of suicidal people then, in the United Kingdom it seems likely that such deliberations would draw upon the case law of the Bolam versus Frien Hospital Management Committee (1957). This appears to be made even more problematic in determining what is the 'right' course of action given that there is wide variation in what would constitute 'good and/or appropriate standards of care' and due to the absence of existing case law featuring the actions or inactions of psychiatric (or any other) nurses. On a related note, on referring to the case of a husband who wished to assist in the requested suicide of his terminally ill wife, the United Kingdom Department of Health (2005) note that:

> 'The Director of Public Prosecutions did not have the power to give an undertaking that he would not consent to prosecute the husband of a terminally-ill woman if he helped his wife to commit suicide. Following an unsuccessful appeal, Mrs Pretty took her case to the European Court of Human Rights (Application no. 2346/02), where judgement went against her on 29 April 2002. Mrs Pretty died unaided on 12 May 2002.'

Thus, it is entirely understandable if practitioners err on the side of caution when making decisions on this issue, for fear of repercussions, criminal prosecution and reprisals from their professional registrative body.

Professional Codes of Conduct: Clear and precise directions?

In these circumstances, practitioners inevitably turn to the Codes of Professional Conduct and Codes of Ethics in the hope they that will offer clear, unambiguous and non-contradictory guidance to their decision making. However, attempting to adhere to Professional Codes of Ethics and/or International Codes of Ethics as a means to guide one's practice, does not always provide easy answers. As with many other ethical dilemmas in healthcare, in the case of assisted suicide it appears difficult, if not impossible to adhere to all the standards/rules at the same time and apply these with equal gusto and fervor. Inevitably, one has to adjudicate between two or more, sometimes conflicting standards/rules and make judicious choices between them. Here, the authors demonstrate these sometimes conflicting standards/rules in the case of assisted suicide by drawing on the principle of respect for autonomy and at the same time the principles of beneficence and non-maleficence (Beauchamp & Childress 1994).

The authors begin with the example of 'irrational' suicide, and here in referring to irrational suicide we are referring to those cases where a person's affect and/or constricted thoughts have ruled out any other options. Furthermore, it refers to cases where intervention from the mental healthcare services could bring about a change of heart; it refers to those cases where there is only a temporary desire to die. In such cases it might be imprudent to respect the suicidal person's right to autonomy since it is quite probable that his/her autonomy is already compromised. As a result the person's decision to commit suicide is not a fully informed choice; it is a 'Hobson's choice' forced upon them by their constricted thoughts, affect and particular world view at that moment in time. In such cases it appears to be reasonable (if not to be required) for the practitioner to adjudicate more towards non-maleficence and beneficence and adopt a paternalistic stance and prevent the person's suicide. While recognizing the breach of the person's individual human rights, the authors are comfortable with this course of action in some (many) circumstances (hence our Relativist approach). Even though this means the authors temporarily assume 'ownership' of another's body and prevent the suicide. In some of our cases of acting in this way, the authors have the 'evidence' of feedback and thanks from people in these circumstances. It may be worthy of note that at the time that the person's liberty and freedom was temporarily removed, the authors may not have had the thanks of the person; the subsequent thanks occurred *ex post facto.*

Perhaps an alternative response is indicated if the practitioner understands the person's decision to end their own life, and what is more regards this as rational, for example, a person who meets the criteria as specified by Speijer and Diekstra (1980) or Werth (1996). In these situations, would it be prudent and appropriate for the practitioner to intervene and prolong life, because this could/would then amount to prolonging the person's suffering and thus violating the ethical code of conduct of beneficence and non-malfecience? Alternatively, if the practitioner intervenes to assist the person with his/her suicide then this would be upholding and even maybe championing the person's right to autonomy; it would be respecting the person's sacrosanct human rights and some would argue, respecting the individual's personhood. The authors stated earlier that they are comfortable with, in some circumstances, temporarily assuming 'ownership' of another's body and preventing suicide, and in support of that, they have the 'evidence' of feedback and thanks from these people – *ex post facto.*

Yet the authors wonder if they have the same thanks from those for whom they prolonged their suffering? One day perhaps, we will know. Rather fittingly, given their undoubted contributions to this debate, we leave the last word to Maris and to Werth and Holdwick:

> *'Sometimes we just need to die, not to be kept alive to suffer pointlessly, and we deserve to be helped in such instances'*
>
> Maris et al 2000

> *'We do a disservice to our clients if we do not prepare ourselves to deal with these issues with them, or, at least, know to whom we can refer them so that they can receive the services they need.'*
>
> Werth and Holdwick 2003, p 533

Chapter 11

Suicide 'Survivors', Reciprocity and Recovery: Issues around Survivors as Therapeutic Agents in the Care of Other Suicidal People

John Cutcliffe, Chris Stevenson and Frank Campbell

'When I lost my husband, I felt so alone. Now as a member of the LOSS Team, I know that I can offer something to new survivors that was unavailable to me during my initial grief. Whenever I hear them ask, 'Kitty, what did you do?' I know that my presence has transcended my role as a responder and become personal as 'survivor to survivor.'
Baton Rouge Crisis Intervention Center website, recovered 2005

CHAPTER CONTENTS

INTRODUCTION

We have stated earlier in this book that the World Health Organization (2002) declares there are over one million suicides world-wide each year. This alone is a startling statistic, but when one considers the wide-spread and far reaching effects that each individual suicide can have, the impact of suicide as a global health problem is even more obvious. As a result, the authors believe it would be remiss to produce a book that focuses on caring for suicidal people without giving some attention and focus to those affected by suicide. However, identifying precisely who are those people who are affected by suicide is no simple task. Accordingly, we begin this chapter by examining the literature regarding this matter. This is followed by examining the growth and development of the suicide survivor 'movement'. Together with identifying and defining suicide survivors, these two matters provide important context for the rest of the issues discussed in the chapter. We follow this brief overview by examining and contributing to the debate concerning the alleged differences in the nature of suicide bereavement when compared to other forms of bereavement. After this, we look at the current pressing research issues within this substantive area.

Given that this is not a generic suicidology textbook and is a book concerned with how one can provide care to suicidal people, we draw this chapter to a close by exploring the possible ways that suicide survivors might work with suicide attempters; these processes are perhaps captured by the notion of moving from anguish to activism and we draw upon testimonies to illustrate these arguments. The authors believe that thus far, as an academe of suicidologists, we have yet to fully embrace the huge potentially therapeutic contribution that some suicide survivors might make in terms of both suicide prevention programs and 'postvention' work with suicide attempters.

DEFINITIONS OF SUICIDE SURVIVORS

Exactly who are suicide survivors? How far reaching is the effect or influence of a suicide death? These are important and yet, hitherto incompletely answered questions. As a community of suicidologists we need more sophisticated and sensitive means to determine how many people can be identified or defined as a 'suicide survivor'. In a similar way to the absence of universally accepted definitions of suicide, there is a related absence of a contemporary, universally accepted or 'standard' definition for a 'suicide survivor'. Interestingly though, together with colleagues, former president of the American Association of Suicidology, Professor David Jobes (Jobes et al 2000, p 538) declared that this lack of an accepted definition is not surprising: 'In our view, no-one can externally or arbitrarily define who is a survivor and who is not a survivor; there can be no rigid or strict definition of the term'.

This absence has not prevented scholars from attempting to address related epidemiological questions. A relatively early, and not necessarily empirically based estimate, posited that there would be at least six people intimately affected by each suicide (McIntosh 1996). Alternatively, it should be noted that 28 people (unique to the deceased) who had a relationship with the deceased, have sought treatment at one crisis centre following suicide

(Campbell 1997, Campbell & Cataldie 2003). Perhaps the apparent disparity in these figures might be explained by recognizing that these two 'approaches' for calculating the figures' focus on two populations. The 6-1 figure as espoused by McIntosh suggests society's view of who 'ought to be impacted by suicide' and such estimates repeatedly suggest that ratio is limited to the next of kin of the deceased. Indeed, the term survivor comes from the obituary which often follows the name of the deceased with 'and is survived by' where only next of kin are listed. Whereas the larger number of 28, as espoused by Campbell and colleagues, declares that many relationships may be impacted to the degree that treatment for that loss is sought. The variety of relationships to the deceased who do seek help suggests that it is virtually impossible to predict who will and will not have long-term negative impact by a suicide.

As a result, contemporary views suggest that these early calculations are likely to have under-estimated the extent of the problem. According to the American Foundation for Suicide Prevention (2003) and the National Institute of Mental Health (2003) well-designed epidemiological studies are clearly needed to determine how many survivors there are, what their characteristics are, and what they need. Clearly, in order for such epidemiological study to have a high degree of accuracy, it is prefaced by some conceptual work to define the population, and when one considers the remarks of Jobes et al (2000), the problem becomes apparent. Part of the problem herein is perhaps identifying when a connection, relationship or 'tie' exists and when it does not. However, it is likely, if not inevitable, that the presence and experience of such relationships are likely to be qualitative phenomena; they are likely to be social constructs and thus not necessarily amenable to quantification. For example, the suicidal death of a student within a University 'ripples' around the entire institution and can effect other students, faculty and staff; irrespective of whether or not there was a direct 'tie' or connection with the deceased (e.g. taught by certain professors, shared classes with certain students, or belonged to certain student groups). The American Foundation for Suicide Prevention (2003) and the National Institute of Mental Health (2003) point out that recent attempts in this area have focused on identifying persons who have known someone who has died by suicide. However, such conceptualizations will not include the innocent by-stander, maid, or first-responder that may witness the suicide or discover the body of someone following the suicide of someone unknown to them. Accordingly, and considering the 'University suicide death' above, the large majority of people who could very well be affected by the suicide are unlikely to have the quantifiable tie 'known to the person who died by suicide' as defined by some epidemiologists. It becomes evident that defining someone as a survivor of a suicide may actually be a phenomenologically defined 'state'; it is perhaps best defined by the individual's own response (or indeed lack of response) to the suicide. This approach embraces that not everyone will be negatively impacted and for those that are, services can be extended and not be limited to society's assumptions of who 'ought to be impacted'.

One further note that needs including here is the concept of clinicians as suicide survivors. The stress of working clinically with suicidal people has been well documented (Barker & Cutcliffe 1999, Campbell 2006, Cutcliffe & Barker 2002, Hamel-Bissel 1985) and the unfortunate truth of the clinical evidence is that, despite the best efforts of these clinicians, some of the suicidal people receiving care will go on to complete suicide; either during their formal care episode or within the first year after discharge. Such is the incidence that Jobes and Berman (1993) found that approximately one half of psychiatrists and one quarter of psychologists will lose at least one person to suicide during the course of their careers. (Interestingly, despite their high level of contact with suicidal people, the authors could find no such data pertaining to P/MH nurses. One could thus extrapolate that P/MH nurses are also likely to be affected, and given the larger numbers involved, may actually represent a larger problem.) In addition to the stress of caring for suicidal people, the stress of losing a suicidal person is understandably worse given the sense of 'failure' that often occurs in such situations. Jobes et al (2000) provide a useful summary of the effects that have been reported in clinicians who have lost a suicidal client, these include:

- High levels of intrusive thoughts relating to patient suicide;
- Avoidance of situations that might remind the clinician of suicide;
- Stress levels roughly equivalent to bereaved patients;
- Self-blame and guilt, particularly about their role in the suicidal person's care;
- Loss of confidence in their professional competence;
- Fear of 'losing face' or standing with professional colleagues;
- Fear of possible malpractice suits from relatives;
- A refusal to 'treat' or work with other suicidal people.

'Positive reactions' include becoming more cautious and vigilant about possible risks of suicide in future clients and improving their suicide prevention skills. Given this documented list of reactions, it is logical to include clinicians as possible suicide survivors. Clinician survivors are also caught in a confusing set of rules and suggestions over how to respond to family questions following the suicide of a patient (Campbell 2006). In the United States, several jurisdictions are developing 'Apology Laws' to allow the clinician to express a statement of condolence without that statement being used as a declaration of liability and then used against the physician in a wrongful death suit (Campbell 2006). Although such a normal response to death of a patient and the offer to help the family in their grief is quite acceptable in most countries, it is often restricted in the United States by professional associations, and malpractice insurance carriers (Campbell 2006). All of these factors contribute to the mixed approaches that are offered survivors by physicians and how they approach their own conflicts following the suicide of someone in their care.

THE GROWTH OF THE SUICIDE SURVIVOR 'MOVEMENT'

Recognition of the bereavement response to suicide and subsequent attention to the needs associated with this experience is a relatively new phenomenon. The comparative lack of empirical enquiry lead Jobes et al (2000, p 540) to state: 'it is remarkable to note that even though suicide has been studied for many years by sociologists and mental health scholars, little direct attention was paid to suicide survivorship until early 1960s'.

Despite the significant advances that have been made, suicide still has a substantial stigma attached to it. In addition, as we pointed out in the previous chapter, because suicide is perceived (by some) as an undesirable act or event, the same people will thus insist on holding someone or something responsible for it (Szasz 1985, 1990). In other words, when suicides occur, there is a need to apportion blame, there is a need to hold someone accountable, and an examination of legal and social responses to suicide throughout history suggest that all too often, the person or persons blamed were the family and other 'suicide survivors'. Jobes et al (2000) describe how with the changing legal and societal perspectives of suicide, blame for suicide began to decline and a corresponding increased recognition of the particular needs of suicide survivors emerged. Equally importantly, not only were survivors able to receive help for their not insignificant needs, and shed the shackles of societal blame, but at the same time the therapeutic contribution that such survivors can make was recognized and preliminary attempts made to mobilize it. The authors believe that this is an overwhelmingly logical and positive development, yet at the same time, one that is in its infancy and has yet to realize the full healing potential that exists. We return to this point later in the chapter.

DIFFERENT PROCESS AND EXPERIENCES? THE DEBATE *APROPOS* SUICIDE BEREAVEMENT AS DISSIMILAR FROM OTHER FORMS OF BEREAVEMENT

According to Jordan (2001), the debate of whether or not suicide bereavement is different from other forms of bereavement has important theoretical and clinical implications. While the authors of this chapter view Jordan's arguments concerning the nature of suicide bereavement as having a compelling quality and cogency, we are somewhat uncomfortable with the whole endeavor to standardize, homogenize, and subsequently quantify the experience of bereavement; particularly if scholars are trying to apply nomothetic, universal law based 'truths' to what is indisputably and incontrovertibly a human experience, and thus inherently unique. While there may be commonalities in the observable elements of many bereavement reactions, or even some commonalities in the process, the personalized, lived experiences, are as individual as snowflakes or one's finger prints. They all share the same basic structure or form, they all have similar characteristics, but they retain their uniqueness. Interestingly, in testimony provided by survivors of suicide, we see the same expressions:

> 'No two people will ever grieve the same way, with the same intensity or for the same duration. It is important to understand this basic truth. Only then can we accept our own manner of grieving and be sensitive to another's response to loss. Only then are we able to seek out the nature of support we need for our own personalized journey back to wholeness and be able to help others on their own journey.'
>
> Baton Rouge Crisis Intervention Center, recovered 2005

For some health-focused scientists, there is a comfort in operating only within nomothetic (universal law) based 'truths' and philosophies/methodologies that embrace such thinking (e.g. positivistic research) – and here we recognize that such researchers often have to bridge and operate within both the medical and social science discourses. While the authors of this book do not wish to decry the contribution to the suicidology academe that such research has made, we do however, recognize its limitations. We have already highlighted the need for methodological pluralism in chapter three. Furthermore, in her insightful paper, Hutchinson (2000, p 506) points out that, within some emerging fields of health/social science, during the 1970s and up to the mid 1980s: 'a time of physics envy prevailed'.

Such a widespread pre-occupation led Munhall (1982, p 177) to state: 'The assumption was that human meaning and behaviour are orderly, lawful, predictable and countable'. And consequently: 'Nursing asserted the similarity of the physical and psychosocial worlds and, in so doing, quantified everything, including clients' beliefs about chemotherapy, parents' experiences with handicapped children, and attitudes towards death'.

It is thus not entirely surprising then that some scholars still wish to quantify and standardize bereavement reactions. Yet as it is pointed out in the words of those who have actually experienced and endured a suicide bereavement:

> *'Not understanding the individuality of grief could complicate and delay whatever grief we might experience from our own loss. It could also influence us, should we attempt to judge the grieving of others – even those we might most want to help.'*
>
> Baton Rouge Crisis Intervention Center, recovered 2005

It should be acknowledged that some researchers have made the argument that there is no empirical evidence to support the assertion that suicide bereavement is more difficult than other forms of bereavement (Cleiren & Diekstra 1995, McIntosh 1993, van der Wal 1989); and here we see that the problem becomes more awkward, given the associated debate around what constitutes evidence and what is empirical evidence. McIntosh (1993) continues to conclude that, after two years, there are few observed differences in suicide bereavement reactions when compared to other types of bereavement reaction. The authors of this book do not doubt the veracity of these claims (and reviews), they do, however, believe that the 'answer' to this question cannot be uncovered using quantitative methods alone and to limit our research activity will only provide incomplete findings; findings of limited theoretical and clinical usefulness. The authors embrace the views posited by Jordan (2001, p 92) namely: 'while acknowledging that it shares many elements common to other forms of loss, . . . bereavement after suicide is sufficiently distinct to merit additional research and specialized clinical services for most suicide survivors'.

Here we offer a summary of Jordan's main points (for a far more thorough and complete review of the relevant theoretical and empirical literature see Jordan 2001).

- While current quantitative studies may have produced equivocal findings regarding the alleged differences between suicide bereavement and other forms of bereavement, (and there exists some well designed studies of these designs that do indicate key differences, see Bailley et al 1999) there is considerable and consistent evidence that the qualitative or thematic aspects of bereavement appear to be different after suicide.

■ Suicide survivors, because of the obvious and different nature of suicide bereavement (e.g. a suicide death is self-inflicted), survivors have different questions around meaning making, or making sense of the death.

■ Suicide survivors have particular issues with self-blame, guilt and responsibility for the death. Survivors report feeling that they somehow caused the death through certain actions/inactions, and/or commonly blame themselves for not anticipating the death.

■ Unfortunately, and despite the significant advances that have been made in this area, not least by the suicide survivor movement themselves, suicide STILL retains a high degree of social stigma in many countries/areas, not surprisingly survivors report receiving less understanding, empathy, compassion and support when compared to people experiencing a less stigmatized bereavement.

Jordan's main points of argument are supported regularly and often within individualized accounts of surviving suicide. Flatt (2000), for example, stated:

'Slowly, crushing guilt became tangled in the anger. I felt like a total failure as a mom – that I was somehow responsible for not equipping my son to make good choices. It seemed my fault that he made this final poor choice to end his life rather than change his self-destructive behavior. I spent hours trying to rework my reality in my mind – trying to find answers to questions that had no answers – as though the answers would somehow change the outcome. Like many survivors, 'If only I had, If only I hadn't', and 'Why?' were my constant thought companions.'

More evidence is provided by survivors who have testimony posted on the Baton Rouge Crisis Intervention website – www.brcic.org – (see loss team section of website) Baton Rouge Crisis Intervention Center, recovered, 2005:

'What kind of help do survivors need? One does not 'get over' a suicide. The effects may stabilize, but the loss is forever felt. Personal values and beliefs are shattered. The individual is changed emotionally. Every survivor needs immediate support at the time of the loss. This is generally not available, which complicates bereavement. Most need long-term support best given by other survivors. Some may need individualized or family counseling or medical care. All need help in understanding suicide and what it has done to their lives.'

Perhaps the most obvious issue for survivors is their own preoccupation with suicide as a consequence for themselves. They often report suicide as a risk factor in their future that was not present before their loss (Campbell 2000). This results in foreshortened future and is not seen in other causes of death. For example the sudden and traumatic death of a parent to other causes of death does not generate a legacy issue for children, whereas this is often reported as a fear by children who lose a parent to suicide. Another common consequence of suicide not experienced by other causes of death is the decision to 'protect' the child by telling them the parent did not die by suicide but by a more 'acceptable' cause of death (Cain 2002). This conspiracy of misinformation is not reported in other causes of death. Why would someone tell the child their dad died in a car accident if he died from a heart attack? Such real approaches to misinformation following a death by suicide are quantifiable and yet research has not taken on the task of describing or measuring this phenomenon. Perhaps research that embraces the reality of the survivor's response will be through using quantitative, qualitative and narrative research to study, describe and contribute to this long lasting debate.

CONTEMPORARY EPISTEMOLOGICAL AND RESEARCH ISSUES *APROPOS* SUICIDE SURVIVOR

As testimony to 'how far' the suicide survivor movement has progressed since the 1960s and 1970s, in 2003, two United States government organizations, the American Foundation for Suicide Prevention (AFSP) and the National Institute of Mental Health (NIMH) organized a workshop. (It should be noted that the United States is far in advance of many other countries with respect to suicide survivor movements and associated research/clinical activity.) This workshop occurred, at least in part, as a response to the lobby from the suicide survivors community regarding the critical importance of conducting research on the impact of suicide on survivors, and in response to their concerns about the limited scope of research-derived knowledge about suicide survivorship. Accordingly, a multi-disciplinary panel of clinicians and suicidology researchers/scholars were invited and assembled and these participants had two major goals.

1. Examine, critique and summarize the extant body of research work relating to suicide survivors.
2. Highlight the gaps in the extant body of knowledge and thus indicate specific research that needs to be conducted (in order to help meet the needs of this population). This would also serve as the framework for producing a research agenda for survivors of suicide.

The full details of this workshop can be found at: http://www.afsp.org/survivor/sosworkshop903.htm and http://rarediseases.info.nih.gov/html/workshops/workshops/suicide2003.htm and here we offer a summary of the main points arising. Given the 'newness' of the suicide survivor movement, it cannot be regarded as surprising that only limited extant work was found; and this paucity of research was perhaps one of the key points emerging from this workshop. Similarly, as we have stated previously, methodological and epistemological endeavors in this area cannot be excluded or separated from associated debates *vis a vis* what constitutes credible and useful evidence; and the associated recognition of the need for methodological pluralism and valuing both idiographic (phenomenological, 'case' based) findings in addition to nomothetic (universal law based) findings. Nevertheless, seven areas in which significant gaps in research knowledge exist were identified and each of these has a number of associated research questions that need to be answered. These were summarized as follows, and are covered in more detail below:

- Defining and identifying 'survivors of suicide'.
- The emotional impact of suicide on: individual family members, families as a whole, therapists who were treating individuals who died by suicide and different cultural, racial and ethnic groups.
- The social adjustment of suicide survivors.

- The risk for suicide and other negative outcomes associated with survivorship.
- The role of first responders (e.g. police officers, emergency medical technicians, emergency room personnel, clergy) in working with survivors.
- Interventions for suicide survivors.
- Methodological and ethical issues in suicide survivor research

Also, additional issues/areas were highlighted in which there has been no systematic examination to date, namely:

- The impact of suicide among gay and lesbian survivors.
- The impact/effects on persons who have lost multiple family members to suicide.

The impact of suicide on family functioning and suicide risk

As we have already covered the issue of defining and identifying 'Survivors of suicide' previously in this chapter, here we consider the impact of suicide on family functioning and suicide risk. Several studies have focused on the emotional responses of individual family members to a suicide. What is noticeabley absent, however, are studies that examine the impact of suicide on the family as a whole. Important questions need to be asked about if and how the suicide of a family member affects family stability and functioning. Interesting suggestions for study include whether there are distinguishing characteristics, traits or processes of families who experience greater closeness and connection following the suicide, than those for whom the suicide results in fragmentation and emotional distance. There is a well validated tool (FACES IV, Olsen & Gorrall 2003) for exploring these aspects of family functioning. Such family dynamics are unlikely to occur in isolation; therefore studies should be undertaken to try and understand the role of cultural/theological values in this process.

The social adjustment of suicide survivors

In place of simplistic characterizations of suicide survivors as one homogeneous group who are thus all likely to experience the same bereavement process, future research in this area needs to address the question of what makes some people particularly vulnerable to severe and persistent distress after a loss due to suicide. Research questions need to be asked about if the particular bereavement reaction is a function of the nature and quality of the relationship with the deceased. Important questions need to be asked about the role of social support and 'connectedness' within one's cultural or sub-cultural groups. What are the processes by which such individuals, families and communities adjust, adapt and cope with the suicide? There would also be utility in trying to gain a deeper and more comprehensive understanding of what contributes to promoting and maintaining resilience among survivors of suicide.

The risk for suicide and other negative outcomes associated with survivorship

It was Shneidman's contention that the largest public health problem is neither the prevention of suicide nor the management of suicide attempts, but the alleviation of the effects of stress in the survivors whose lives are forever altered (Shneidman 1973). Similarly, there is a body of work that indicates how experiencing a suicide within one's family can increase the risk of further suicides within that family. While we do have at least two posited theories, the precise mechanism (or more likely mechanisms) of this process are not well understood. Further, we have a limited understanding of the increased risks of people experiencing mental health problems subsequent to a suicide within one's family, though it is ethically and methodologically problematic to attempt to undertake controlled studies to add to the evidence in this area.

Interventions (postventions) for suicide survivors

Edwin Shneidman coined the term 'postvention' to describe appropriate and helpful acts that come after a dire event (Shneidman 1973). As previously cited in this chapter, who qualifies as a survivor has been unclear over the decades; what does seem to persist is the notion that survivors who do get help report better outcomes. However, very little research evidence exists to inform clinicians (and others) about how we might best offer support to and help suicide survivors. The 'interventions' we do have are currently lacking in empirical underpinnings, and thus the matter of knowing how to help survivors of suicide remains pressing; although, it should be noted that a number of narrative accounts might offer valuable insight into this issue. A limited amount of research, with encouraging findings, exists regarding specific 'postvention' interventions; though clearly more is needed as it is unlikely that 'one size will fit all'; that one postvention intervention will be discovered that can be universally applied to all survivors of suicide.

The anecdotal and narrative-based evidence emerging from suicide-bereavement support groups is consistent in showing that such groups are considered to be, and found to be, helpful by many survivors. Though for some, questions have been asked about this evidence as the data have been obtained from small, non-representative samples. A number of studies undertaken with additional interventions have produced equivocal findings, and again for some, are of limited value give the size of samples used and the due to lack of appropriate control or comparison groups. Interestingly, just as with care of the suicidal person, it has yet to be determined what constitutes 'treatment as usual' for survivors of suicide or indeed if this is a useful term.

The role of first responders (e.g. police officers, emergency medical technicians, emergency room personnel, clergy) in working with survivors

We know very little about the impact of 'first responders', including emergency room providers, clergy and funeral directors, on survivors' emotional responses and adjustment.

Methodological and ethical issues in suicide survivor research

Research in and around the formal area of 'suicide survivors' is replete with a number of significant methodological challenges. For some these challenges include, but are not restricted to:

- the low base rate of suicide
- finding less biased samples

- conducting randomized experimental trials of interventions with carefully defined and selected comparison groups
- the development and use of valid and reliable measures of specified outcomes (e.g., severity of survivor distress, psychological closeness between the survivor and the individual who died by suicide)
- the challenges involved in studying subgroups with unique issues.

For others, some of these methodological challenges are overcome by embracing a multi-method approach to knowledge generation; by accepting idiographic case-related findings in addition to nomothetic findings and by recognizing that these experiences of surviving suicide are *phenomenologically defined* (our emphasis).

MOVING FROM ANGUISH TO ACTIVISM: POSTVENTION IN THE FORM OF CARING FOR SUICIDAL OTHERS

If one regards the view that any suicide bereavement is a phenomenologically unique experience (while sharing elements that are common to other forms of loss), to be axiomatic, then it follows that the process of surviving suicide (or recovering from suicide) is similarly unique. As a result it is unlikely, if not highly improbable, that one process of facilitating 'recovery' from suicide will be appropriate for, therapeutic for, or even necessary for all suicide survivors. As a result, in no way would the authors of this book purport that one can identify an 'intervention' or process of healing/recovery that will be applicable, useful or meaningful to each and every survivor or suicide. Nevertheless, there may be experiences and processes that have utility and transferability across individualized suicide bereavement experiences, in the same way that some interventions and/or processes have been found to have utility across other bereavement experiences. For example, the need for adaptation to reality of the loss, the bereft individual being able to experience a sense of 'distance' or 'freedom' from the deceased, the importance of experiencing and 'facing up to' the emotional pain associated with the loss. (see Anderson & Dimond 1995, Kato & Mann 1999, Kavanagh 1990, Lendrum & Syme 1992, Lloyd 1992, Martocchio 1985, Parkes 1980, Parkes & Brown 1972, Prigerson et al 1995, Raphael et al 1993, Raphael & Middleton 1987, Schut et al 1997, Scruby & Sloan 1989, Tschudin 1997, Worden 1988). As a result, this section of the chapter focuses on processes that have been found to be therapeutic and beneficial for suicide survivors and in addition, offers preliminary arguments around the concept of 'survivors as helpers of people who have made a serious attempt on their lives'.

What works?

It is necessary to preface this section by acknowledging that very little 'empirical' evidence exists so far that demonstrates what does and what does not work for suicide survivors. An examination of the relevant literature appears to indicate that the only suicide survivor 'intervention' that has undergone a systematic evaluation of an Active Postvention Model (APM) is the LOSS Team programme emanating out of The Baton Rouge Crisis

Intervention Centre, Louisiana, developed by Dr Frank Campbell, past president of the American Association of Suicidology (Campbell et al 2004). (We use the term 'intervention' cautiously as there is not one single intervention.) This unique programme, termed Local Outreach to Suicide Survivors (LOSS) was deigned for those who have lost a loved one to suicide; it was designed to offer immediate support to survivors as close to the time of death as possible. The programme is described as a 'first response team' and consists of survivor volunteers and centre staff, who in response to a suicide in the local area, will arrive at the 'scene' of the suicide in order to offer resources, support, and sources of hope to the newly bereaved (www.brcic.org Baton Rouge Crisis Intervention Center website, recovered 2005). The authors firmly believe that this programme is the first example of the huge therapeutic potential that exists in combining formal healthcare resources with suicide survivors; a potential which is hitherto unexplored and under-valued. Interestingly, the evaluatory evidence in relation to the program makes compelling reading.

> 'I cannot express how much help the Baton Rouge Crisis Intervention Center and all of the wonderful people there have been since my father's suicide a few weeks ago. They were a wonderful source of support the day of the incident, and were at our house within 15 minutes of the call letting us know that we were not alone and they were there for us, 24-hours a day. This meant more to us as survivors than anything else. Please see that this service is made available to everyone, in all States, for it has helped us through the most difficult thing a person could ever have to face. We appreciate all they did, and are still doing, and feel truly blessed to have such wonderful support.'

And

> 'This service of the LOSS Team has been the turning point in my ability to cope with this issue. The guidance and understanding I've gained have shown me how to get through these times. I am very happy to have this chance to understand and learn how to cope. The Crisis Center is very important to me. I hope others will be able to learn, like I have, how this service is needed. Thanks for being there for my family and myself.'
> Baton Rouge Crisis Intervention Center website, recovered 2005

As valuable as this LOSS programme is, the authors of this book suggest that there may be additional areas and/or situations where suicide survivors might make a further therapeutic contribution; and that is within the domain of working with people who have made a serious attempt at suicide (for example, the people who participated as participants in the reported research). Furthermore, we believe that such endeavours could have reciprocal therapeutic value for both parties. It strikes the authors of this chapter that such models of care may be analogous to encouraging people who are on the recovery from substance/alcohol misuse (or currently engaged in harm reduction), to work as 'health promoters' and with others who have substance misuse problems. There is a significant and growing body of evidence that refers to the value of having 'recovered' substance users speak to current users. Indeed, according to this body of work, we see that the most powerful testimony and with that, infusion of hope for people with substance misuse problems comes from others who have gone through the same/similar experience and recovered/survived. There are clear messages conveyed here of: 'Look at me, I never thought I could do it – but I did! Recovery is possible. If I can do it – you can too! There is hope for you; I was once where you were are now.' There are existing examples of former users acting in health promotion roles, for example, these (and we consider them to be brave and generous) individuals will speak to groups of school children.

Another example of this largely unexplored therapeutic potential that may reside in encouraging suicide survivors to engage in proactive care of others is that of the 'Suicide Anonymous' (SA) group that was begun by a psychiatrist and self identified 'serial attempter' in Memphis, Tennessee. Dr Ken Tullis proposed the use of the 12-step model and created a group of attempters who support each other in living the way 'alcoholics' support sobriety.

Furthermore, some of the literature pertaining to suicidal young men and their particular needs speaks of this idea. One of the things these young men identify is that they would like to be able to talk to a friend – but cannot. Such is the societal and cultural constructs of what it is to be a (young) man is that discussing one's problems with one's peer group is often not a viable option. (i.e. not macho, don't want to be 'a downer'). This group are similarly reluctant to talk with or to formal services; this is too scary (i.e. fears around confidentiality, strangers, and associated stigma). Accordingly, it might be that that speaking to another young man who has 'been there' might be a more acceptable form of help. (The authors are pleased to report that they have research into this issue ongoing in Ireland.)

The authors are aware that, for some, this suggestion may appear to be unsafe for all parties concerned and we need to address some of these concerns. Firstly, it is axiomatic that being involved in the care of other suicidal people may not be suitable or appropriate for all suicide survivors. No suicide survivor should be in any way forced or coerced into such activity; their involvement would need to be a pro-active matter of choice. Secondly, any such involvement of a suicide survivor would need to occur at a time/place in the survivor's own recovery when he/she is in good enough emotional shape to deal with whatever comes up for. There appears to be a logical assumption that being involved too early in one's own recovery would possibly be counterproductive. Thirdly, suicide survivors would need to operate with the appropriate level of clinical supervision. Not clinical supervision as a form of performance monitoring, but supervision *apropos* psychotherapy and/or P/MH nursing in order that they get the necessary emotional support. (See Cutcliffe and Lowe (2005) for a recent exploration of the key differences in conceptualization and resultant practice of clinical supervision.) Fourthly, suicide survivors operating in this way should also be provided with an additional 'safety net' of support services; should they feel the need to re-examine some of their own reaction/response/issues. Fifthly, it might be prudent for suicide survivors always to work in partnership with a trained, professional mental health practitioner (all five of these points are present and required for invitation to join the Baton Rouge LOSS Team). Since 1999 when the LOSS Team approach began being the primary way of responding to suicides in their service area, the average number of days between the death and seeking help at the Baton Rouge Crisis Center has gone from 4.5 years to less than 44 days (Campbell 2006, Campbell et al 2004). The next research will be to determine if coming in sooner had a positive impact on those who received a loss team visit at the time of death. Even though the abundance of anecdotal evidence supports an Active Postvention Model, it will be necessary to verify what benefits are derived from the visit from a survivor while the body is still present. This Active Postvention Model (APM) has been adopted as the national model in Singapore, over a dozen communities in the United States as well as other communities and countries around the world. The installation of hope that the newly bereaved will survive from contact by another survivor at the scene of the suicide is one of the most often reported motivators' survivors who seek treatment report. In addition many group members in Baton Rouge declare (as a personal goal of their own) they hope one day to be on the LOSS Team so they can do for someone else what was done for them.

Further support for the notion of suicide survivors as potential therapeutic agents for other suicidal people is perhaps found in the literature referring to the 'Wounded Helper' (see Hawkins & Shohet 2000). Expressed in its simplest form, this notion suggests that very few (if any?) mental health care practitioners are free from their own issues, psychological angst, or even psychological pain. Yet the presence (and influence) of these intrapersonal dynamics does not prevent the practitioner from offering care to others. Further, accepting the legitimacy of psychoanalytical (psychodynamic) theories of interpersonal helping, these intrapersonal issues will influence the therapeutic encounter through projection, transference/counter-transference and the practitioner's defence mechanisms. (Here, the authors acknowledge that, for some, these terms are interchangeable and for others they are not.) At the same time, various intra- and interpersonal mechanisms and processes exist in order to enable the practitioner to go on working with clients (e.g. receiving and engaging in clinical supervision, receiving one's own therapy, informal support from peers/colleagues). This issue is captured beautifully by Hawkins and Shohet (2000, p 192):

> 'The middle ground entails being on the path of facing our own shadow, our own fear, hurt, distress and helplessness, and taking responsibility for ensuring that we practise what we preach. This means managing our own support system, finding friends and colleagues who will not just reassure us but also challenge our defenses, and finding a supervisor or supervision group who will not collude in trying to see who can be most potent with ways of curing the client, but will attend to how we are stuck in relating to the full truth of those with whom we work.'

Accordingly, while accepting that the involvement of suicide survivors in care of other suicidal people may be problematic, and may at times even give rise to identification issues, mechanisms and processes currently exist in facilitating professional practitioners to deal with their own material, and the authors of this book suggest that similar support systems could be put in place for suicide survivors. It is clear that each of us as formal or informal practitioners or helpers of suicidal people does not have to be 'free from any sense of psychological angst' in order to be able to work therapeutically and successfully. As a result the authors would argue that personal experience of suicide (i.e. being a suicide survivor) should not rule that person out from offering help to other suicidal people; indeed it may well be that such individuals are very well placed to offer help.

Reciprocal healing?

A further argument for considering the role of some suicide survivors in the care of suicidal people goes to the idea of reciprocal healing or reciprocal gain. Even a cursory examination of the narrative accounts that proliferate in the suicide survivor literature will show that some (many?) survivors (e.g. Iris Bolton, Linda Flatt and Teri Wise) transform their personal experience of suicide (or indeed personal suicide attempt) into something that can help others. Powerful and compelling testimony is included on the LOSS website:

> 'When I lost my husband, I felt so alone. Now as a member of the LOSS Team, I know that I can offer something to new survivors that was unavailable to me during my initial grief. Whenever I hear them ask, 'Kitty, what did you do?' I know that my presence has transcended my role as a responder and become personal as 'survivor to survivor.'

> Baton Rouge Crisis Intervention Center website, recovered 2005

Whereas another suicide survivor states:

> 'The months following my father's death were unbearable. I was overwhelmed by emotions and thoughts that I didn't understand. My confusion was leading me to the exact place my father was when he decided to end his life. Luckily, I stumbled upon the Survivors of Suicide Support Group. Imagine my surprise to meet other people with losses to suicide – even other people my age who had lost a parent to suicide! As I dragged myself out of that lonely pit of hopelessness, I felt sorry for those who did not have such support. As a member of the LOSS team, I know the difference that comes with immediate support. The new survivors I meet at the scene don't have to stumble across the help that can mean the difference between life and death. They don't have to struggle for months or even years. Help and support and hope are right there with them at that same moment they're feeling ravaged and alone and confused. I hope that one day every new survivor will get the immediate response that they deserve.'

Similarly, Flatt (2000) offers the following remarks about her own 'transformation':

> 'But I soon became aware that suicide bereavement was a part of who I was. It was up to me to decide how I would incorporate that experience into my life.'

And:

> 'Sharing my pain with others who are also broken-hearted by a suicide death –and watching the victories come from the struggles in the group – have been the gifts that Iris Bolton promised me in her book, My Son, My Son'.

Flatt concludes:

> 'For over six years I have traveled from the healing path to the survivor support path – and on to the prevention advocacy path. It is a path I am now comfortable with, because I have worked through my feelings of guilt and responsibility for my son's death.'

Looking at Linda's testimony, it strikes the authors that perhaps sometimes the survivor might be unaware of the potential healing and therapeutic power that could reside in such activity for themselves. Indeed, Linda Flatt and others declare that, at first, the idea of helping others as a suicide survivor held no interest (and much fear) for them. Yet, in receiving the appropriate and adequate support themselves, the reciprocal gain or reciprocal healing was encountered. In helping others, Linda and others were thus engaging in their own healing journey. It is important to point out that this would not be the primary reason for engaging in helping others, but there is a growing body of anecdotal evidence which attests to these reciprocal therapeutic gains, to the added meaning brought to lives of suicide survivors that helping others in similar situations brings about.

References

Adam R, Tille S, Pollock L 2003 Person first: what people with enduring mental disorders value about Community Psychiatric Nurses and CPN services. Journal of Psychiatric and Mental Health Nursing 10:203–212

Alderfer B 1972 Existence, relatedness, and human growth: human needs in organisational settings. Free Press, Oxford

Aldridge D 1998 Suicide: the tragedy of hopelessness. Jessica Kingsley, London

Althscul A 1972 Patient–nurse interaction: a study of interaction patterns in acute psychiatric wards. Churchill Livingstone, Edinburgh

Altschul A 1997 A personal view of psychiatric nursing. In: Tilley S (ed) The mental health nurse: views of practice and education. Blackwell Science, London, p 1–14

Alvarez A 1970 The savage God. Random House, New York

Anderson KL, Dimond MF 1995 The experience of bereavement in older adults. Journal of Advanced Nursing 22:308–315

Anderson M, Standen P, Noon J 2003 Nurses' and doctors' perceptions of young people who engage in suicidal behaviour: a contemporary grounded theory analysis. International Journal of Nursing Studies 40(6):587–597

Aquinas T 1945 Basic writings of Thomas Aquinas. Randon House, New York

Asberg M, Traskman L, Thorien P 1976 5-HIAA in cerebrospinal fluid: a biochemical suicide prediction? Archives of General Psychiatry 33:1193–1197

Asberg M, Nordstrom P, Traskman-Bendz L 1990 Cerebrospinal fluid studies in suicide: an overview. Annals of the New York Academy of Sciences 487:243–255

Avis M, Bond M, Arthur A 1994 Patient satisfaction and the management of outpatient consultation. Unpublished Report, University of Nottingham, Nottingham

Bagley C 1991 Poverty and suicide among native Canadians: a replication. Psychological Reports 69(1):149–150

Bagley C 1992 Changing profiles of a typology of youth suicide in Canada. Canadian Journal of Public Health 83(2):169–170

Bagley C, Ramsey RR 1989 Attitudes towards suicide, religious values and suicidal behaviour: evidence from a community survey. In: Diekstra R et al (eds) Suicide and its prevention: the role of attitude and imitation. Brill, Leiden

Bailley SE, Kral MJ, Dunham K 1999 Survivors of suicide do grieve differently: empirical support for a common sense proposition. Suicide and Life-Threatening Behavior 29: 256–271

Barker P 1997 A meta-theory of psychiatric nursing practice Mental Health Practice 1(4):18–21

Barker P 1999 The philosophy and practice of psychiatric nursing. Churchill Livingstone, Edinburgh

Barker P, Buchanan P 2005 Observation: the original sin of mental health. Journal of Psychiatric and Mental Health Nursing 12:541–549

Barker P, Cutcliffe JR 1999 Clinical risk: a need for engagement not observation. Mental Health Care 2:8–12

Barker P, Cutcliffe JR 2000a Creating a hopeline for suicidal people: a new model for acute sector mental health nursing. Mental Health Care 3(6):190–193

Barker P, Cutcliffe JR 2000b Hoping against hope. Open Mind 101:18–19

Barker P, Walker L 1999 A survey of care practices in acute admission wards. Report submitted to the Northern and Yorkshire Regional Research and Development Committee, University of Newcastle

Barker P, Reynolds B, Stevenson C 1997 The human science basis of psychiatric nursing: theory and practice. Journal of Advanced Nursing 25(4):660–667

Barker P, Jackson S, Stevenson C 1999 What are psychiatric nurses needed for? Developing a theory of essential nursing practice. Journal of Psychiatric and Mental Health Nursing 6(4):273–282

Barnes RA, Ennis J, Schober R 1986 Cohort analysis of Ontario suicide rates 1877–1976. Canadian Journal of Psychiatry 31:208–213

Barraclough B, Bunch J, Nelson P, Sainsbury P 1974 A hundred cases of suicide: clinical aspects. British Journal of Psychiatry 125:355–373

Baton Rouge Crisis Intervention Center website (recovered 2005). http://www.brcic.org/pro_loss.html

Battin MP, Rhodes R, Silvers A (eds) 1998 Physician assisted suicide: expanding the debate. Routledge, London

Beauchamp and Childress 1994 Principles of bio-medical ethics, 3rd edn. Oxford University Press, Oxford

Beautrais AL, Joyce PR, Mulder RT et al 1996 Prevalence and co-morbidity of mental disorders in persons making serious suicide attempts: a case-control study. American Journal of Psychiatry 153:1009–1014

Beck A, Brown G, Berchick R et al 1990 Relationship between hopelessness and ultimate suicide: a replication with psychiatric outpatients. American Journal of Psychiatry 147(2):190–195

Beech P, Normal IJ 1995 Patients' perceptions of the quality of psychiatric nursing care: Findings from a small scale descriptive study. Journal of Clinical Nursing 4:117–123

Beneteau X 1988 Trends in suicide. Canadian Social Trends 11:22–24

Berman AL, Jones D, Silverman MM 2005 Adolescent suicide: assessment and intervention, 2nd edn. American Psychological Association, Washington DC

Berne E 1964 Games people play. Grove, New York

Bonner RL, Rich AR 1987 High consequences of loneliness: a review of the literature. Journal of American College Health 37:162–167

Bowers L 2001 Response to J Cutcliffe. (28.501) Psychiatric Nursing discussion list. Electronic internet reference.

Bowles N, Dodds P, Hackney D et al 2002 Formal observations and engagement: a discussion paper. Journal of Psychiatric and Mental Health Nursing 9(3):255–260

British Columbia Vital Statistics Agency 2001 Selected vital statistics and health status indicators: one hundred and thirtieth annual report of the BCVSA. BCVSA, Victoria

British Columbia Vital Statistics Agency 2002 Selected vital statistics and health status indicators: one hundred and thirty first annual report of the BCVSA. BCVSA, Victoria

British Medical Association 1998 Euthanasia and physician assisted suicide: do the moral arguments differ? A discussion paper from the BMA's Medical Ethics Department. BMA, London

British Medical Association (recovered 2005) Physician assisted suicide: the law http://www.bma.org.uk/ap.nsf/Content/Physician+assisted+suicide:+The+lw

Brown M, Fowler G 1971 Psychodynamic nursing: a biosocial oreintation. WB Saunders, Philadelphia

Brown M, Fowler G 1979 Psychodynamic nursing: a biosocial orientation. WB Saunders, Philadelphia

Cain AC 2002 Children of suicide: the telling and the knowing. Psychiatry 65(2):124–136

Campbell FR 1997 Changing the legacy of suicide, Suicide and Life-Threatening Behavior 27(4)

Campbell FR 2000 Suicide: an American form of family abuse. New Global Development XVI:88–93.

Campbell FR 2001a Living and working in the canyon of why. Proceedings of the Irish Association of Suicidology 6:96–97

Campbell FR 2001b Changing the legacy of suicide through an active model of postvention. Proceedings of the Irish Association of Suicidology 6:26–29

Campbell FR 2006 Aftermath of suicide: the clinician's role. In: Simon RI, Hales RE (eds) The American psychiatric publishing textbook of suicide assessment and management. American Psychiatric Publishing, Washingtom DC, p 459–476

Campbell FR, Cataldie L 2003 Survivor support teams. Paper presented at the Survivors of Suicide Research Workshop Program, NIMH/NIH Office of Rare Diseases and the American Foundation for Suicide Prevention, Bethesda MD

Campbell FR, Cataldie L, McIntosh J, Millet K 2004 An active postvention program. Crisis 25(1):30–32

Campbell P 2006 Commentary. In: Cutcliffe JR, Ward MF (eds) Key debates in psychiatric/mental health nursing. Elsevier, London, p 272–276

Camus A 1945 The myth of Sisyphus (translated by J O'Brien). Harris Hamilton, London

Canadian Association for Suicide Prevention 2004 Blueprint for a Canadian National Suicide Prevention Strategy. www.suicideprevention.ca

Canadian Psychiatric Association 2004 Limitation of freedom of movement in adult psychiatric units. http://www.cpa-apc.org/publications/position-papers/movement.asp

Cardell R, Pitula CR 1999 Suicidal inpatients' perceptions of therapeutic and non-therapeutic aspects of constant observation. Psychiatric Services 20(8):1066–1070

Caron J, Grenier H, Beguin B 1995 Le suicide en Abitibi-Temiscaminique: donnees epidemiologipues pour le period 1986-1990. Review Canadienne de sante communautaine 14(1):79–101

Carr E, Mann E 2000 Pain. Creative approaches to effective pain management. Palgrave Macmillan, Hampshire

Carrigan JT 1994 The psychosocial need of patient who attempt suicide by overdose. Journal of Advanced Nursing 20:635–642

Centre for Suicide Prevention 2005 Facing the facts: suicide in Canada. Centre for Suicide Prevention, Calgary

Chan PA, Rudman MJ 1998 Paradigms for mental health nursing: fragmentation or integration? Journal of Psychiatric and Mental Health Nursing 5:143–146

Charlton J, Bauer R, Thankore A et al 1987 Unemployment and mortality: a small area analysis. Journal of Clinical Epidemiology and Community Health 41:107–113

Charlton J, Kelly S, Dunnell K et al 1992 Trends in suicide deaths in England and Wales. Population Trends 69:6–10

Charlton J Kelly S, Dunnell K et al 1994a Trends in suicide deaths in England and Wales. In: Jenkins R et al (eds) The prevention of suicide. Department of Health. HMSO, London, p 6–12

Charlton J, Kelly S, Dunnell K et al 1994b Suicide deaths in England and Wales: trends in factors associated with suicide deaths. In: Jenkins R et al (eds) The prevention of suicide. Department of Health. HMSO, London, p 13–21

Cheifetz PN, Posener JK, LaHaye A et al 1987 An epidemiologic study of adolescent suicide. Canadian Journal of Psychology 32:656–659

Clancy K (recovered 2005) David Kelly, British biological weapons expert, commits suicide. The Hill–Chapel Hill Political Review http://www.ibiblio.org/thehill/issues/vol_iii_issue_1/KelliClancy.html

Cleiren M, Diekstra R 1995 After the loss: bereavement after suicide and other types of death. In: Mishara B (ed) The impact of suicide. Springer, New York, p 7–39

Crombie IK 1990 Can changes in unemployment rates explain the recent changes in suicide rates in developed countries? International Journal of Epidemiology 2:412–416

Crook M 2003 Out of the Darkness: teens talk about suicide. Arsenal Pulp Press, Vancouver

Cutcliffe JR 2003 The differences and commonalities between United Kingdom and Canadian Psychiatric/Mental health nursing: a personal reflection. Journal of Psychiatric and Mental Health Nursing 10:255–257

Cutcliffe JR 2004 The inspiration of hope in bereavement counselling. Jessica Kingsley, London

Cutcliffe JR 2005a Towards an understanding of suicide in First Nation Canadians. Crisis: the journal of crisis intervention and suicide prevention 26(3):141–145

Cutcliffe JR 2005b Challenging normative orthodoxies in depression: Huxley's Utopia or Dante's Inferno? Conference proceedings 29th International Congress of the International Academy of Law and Mental Health, Paris, France, July 2005

Cutcliffe JR, Barker P 2002 Considering the care of the suicidal client and the case for 'engagement and inspiring hope' or observations. Journal of Psychiatric and Mental Health Nursing 9(5):611–621

Cutcliffe JR, Lowe L 2005 A comparison of North American and European conceptualisations of clinical supervision. Issues in Mental Health Nursing 26(5):475–488

Cutcliffe JR, McKenna HP 2004 Expert qualitative researchers and the use of audit trails. Journal of Advanced Nursing 45(2):126–133

Cutcliffe JR, Ramcharan P 2002 Leveling the playing field: Considering the 'ethics as process' approach for judging qualitative research proposals. Qualitative Health Research 12(7):1000–1010

Cutcliffe JR, Ward MF 2006 Critiquing nursing research, 2nd edn. Quay Books, London

Cutcliffe JR, Dukintis J, Carberry J 1997 User's views of their continuing care community psychiatric services. International Journal of Psychiatric Nursing Research 3(3): p 382–394

Cutcliffe JR, Butterworth T, Proctor B 2001 Fundamental themes in clinical supervision. Routeledge, London

Davidhizar R, Vance A 1993 The management of the suicidal patient in a critical care unit. Journal of Nursing Management 1:95–102

Davidson L 2003 Book reviews: contemporary perspectives on rational suicide. American Journal of Psychiatry 11:108–109.

Dawson PJ 1997 A reply to Kevin Gournay's 'Schizophrenia: a review of the contemporary literature and implications for mental health nursing theory, practice and education'. Journal of Psychiatric and Mental Health Nursing 4:1–7

Denzin N, Lincoln YS 1994 Introduction: Entering the field of qualitative enquiry In:Denzin N, Lincoln YS (eds) Handbook of Qualitative Research. Sage, London, p 1–14

Department of Health 1990 Health of the nation. HMSO, London

Department of Health 1998a Modernising mental health services: safe, sound and supportive. HMSO, London

Department of Health 1998b Our healthier nation: a contract for health. HMSO, London

Department of Health 1999a National Service Framework for Mental Health. HMSO, London

Department of Health 1999b Safer services – national confidential inquiry into suicides and homicides by people with mental health problems. HMSO, London

Department of Health 2001 Safety first: five year report of the national confidential inquiry into suicide and homicide by people with mental illness HMSO, London

Department of Health 2005 National suicide prevention strategy for England, 2nd Annual Report on progress. HMSO, London

Department of Health (recovered 2005) Human rights case law http://www.dh.gov.uk/PolicyAndGuidance/EqualityAndHumanRights/EqualityAnHumanRightsArticle/fs/en?CONTENT_ID=4054188&chk=S7bmtd

Dickinson K, Mathers N, Newton P, Seager P 1996 Confidential inquiry into deaths by suicide in Sheffield 1993. Clinical Audit Department, Community Health NHS Trust Sheffield, Sheffield

Diekstra R 1992 Suicide and euthanasia Giornale Italiano de Suicidologia 2:71–78

Dodds P, Bowles N 2001 Dismantling formal observation and refocusing nursing activity in acute inpatient psychiatry: a case study. Journal of Psychiatric and Mental Health Nursing 8:173–188

Dooley E 1990 Prison suicide in England and Wales 1972–1987. British Journal of Psychiatry 156:40–45

Douglas JD 1967 The social meanings of suicide. Princeton University Press, Princeton

Duckworth G, McBride H 1996 Suicide in old age: a tragedy of neglect. Canadian Journal of Psychiatry 41:217–222

Duffy D 1995 Out of the Shadows: a study of the special observation of suicidal psychiatric in-patients. Journal of Advanced Nursing 21:944–950

Duffy D 2003 Exploring suicide risk in the therapeutic relationship: a case study approach Nursing Times Research 8(3):185–199

Dunnell K 1994 Epidemiology and trends in suicide in the UK. In: Jenkins R et al (eds) The Prevention of Suicide. HMSO, London

Durkheim E 1951 Suicide: a study in sociology (original work 1897). Free Press, Glencoe IL

Dyck RJ, Newman SC, Thompson AH 1988 Suicide trends in Canada 1956–1981. Homicide Studies 2:46–63

Egan MP 1997 Contracting for safety: a concept analysis. Crisis 18:17–23

Elbeck M, Fecteau G 1990 Improving the validity of measures of patient satisfaction with psychiatric care and treatment. Hospital and Community Psychiatry 41 (9):998–1001

Ellis TE, Ratliff KG 1986 Cognitive characteristics of suicidal and nonsuicidal psychiatric inpatients. Cognitive Therapy and Research 10(6):625–634

Eynan R, Langley J, Tolomiczenko G et al 2002 The association between homelessness and suicidal ideation and behaviours: results of a cross-sectional survey. Suicide and Life-Threatening Behavior 32(4):418–427

Fawcett J, Scheftner W, Clark D et al 1987 Clinical predictors of suicide in patients with major affective disorders: a controlled prospective study American Journal of Psychiatry 144(1):35–40

Feldman R, Eidelman AI, Sirota L, Weller A 2002 Effects of skin-to-skin contact (Kangaroo care) on parenting and infant development in premature infants Peadiatrics 110: 16–26

Flatt L 2000 Reflections of a survivor – from anguish to activism: transcending a suicide loss. Lifesavers Quarterly newsletter from AFSP American Foundation for Suicide Prevention 12(1)

Fletcher RF 1999 The process of constant observation: perspectives of staff and suicidal patients. Journal of sychiatric and Mental Health Nursing 6:9–14

Fonagy P, Bateman AW 2006 Mechanisms of change in mentalization-based treatment of BPD. Journal of Clinical Psychology 62:411–430

Fox AJ, Shewry MC 1988 New longitudinal insights into relationships between unemployment and mortality. Stress Medicine 4:11–19

Frankl V 1959 Man's search for meaning. Hodder & Stoughton, London

Freud A 1949 Aggression in relation to emotional development: normal and pathological. Psychoanalytic Study of the Child 3:37–42

Garnefski N, Diekstra RF, DeHeus P 1992 A population-based survey of the characteristics of high-school students with and without a history of suicidal behaviour. Acta Psychiatrica Scandinavica 86:189–196

Geddes JR, Juszczak E 1995 Period trends in rate of suicide in first 28 days after discharge from psychiatric hospital in Scotland, 1968–92. BMJ 311:357–360

Geddes JR, Juszczak E, O'Brien F, Kendrick S 1997 Suicide in the 12 months after discharge from psychiatric inpatient care, Scotland 1968–92. Journal of Epidemiology and Community Health 51:430–434

Gibbs A 1990 Aspects of communication with people who have attempted suicide. Journal of Advanced Nursing 15:1245–1249

Glaser BG 1978 Theoretical sensitivity: Advances in the methodology of grounded theory. Sociology Press, Mill Valley CA

Glaser BG 1992 Basics of grounded theory analysis: emerging versus forcing Sociology Press, Mill Valley CA

Glaser BG 1998 Doing grounded theory: issues and discussions. Sociology Press, Mill Valley CA

Glaser BG 2001 The grounded theory perspective: conceptualisation contrasted with description. Sociology Press, Mill Valley CA

Glaser BG, Strauss AL 1967 The discovery of grounded theory: strategies for qualitative research. Aldine, Chicago

Goldacre M, Seagroatt V, Hawton K 1993 Suicide after discharge from psychiatric inpatient care. Lancet 342:283–286

Goldney RD 2002 Qualitative and quantitative approaches in Suicidology: commentary. Archives of Suicide Research 6(1):69–73

Goldstein RB, Black DW, Nasrallah A, Winokur G 1991 The prediction of suicide: sensitivity, specificity and predictive value of a multivariate model applied to suicide among 1906 patients with an affective disorder. Archives of General Psychiatry 48:418–422

Gordon D, Alexander DA, Dieztan J 1979 The psychiatric patient: a voice to be heard. British Journal of Psychiatry 135:115–121

Gournay K 1996 Schizophrenia: a review of the contemporary literature and implications for mental health nursing theory, practice and education. Journal of Psychiatric and Mental Health Nursing 3:7–12

Gournay K, Ward M, Thornicroft G et al 1998 Crisis in the capital: inpatient care in inner London. Mental Health Practice 1:10–18

Gray JE, O'Reilly RL 2001 Clinically significant differences among Canadian mental health acts. Canadian Journal of Psychiatry 46:315–321

Gunnell D, Frankel S 1994 Prevention of suicide: aspirations and evidence. British Medical Journal 308:1227–1233

Gunnell DJ, Peters TJ, Kammerling RM, Brooks J 1995 Relation between para suicide, suicide, psychiatric admissions , and socioeconomic deprivation. British Medical Journal 311:226–230

Hamel-Bissel BP 1985 Suicidal casework: assessing nurses' reactions Journal of Psychosocial Nursing and Mental Health Services 23:20–23

Hannigan B, Cutcliffe JR 2002 Challenging contemporary mental health policy: time to assuage the coercion? Journal of Advanced Nursing 35(5):477–484

Harlow HF, Suomi SJ 1970 The nature of love simplified. American Psychologist 25:161–168

Harris EC, Barraclough BM 1998 Suicide as an outcome for mental disorders: a meta-analysis. British Journal of Psychiatry 170:205–228

Hasselback P, Lee KI, Mao Y et al 1991 The relationship of suicide rates to socisodemographic factors in Canadian census divisions. Canadian Journal of Psychiatry 36:655–659

Hawkins P, Shohet R 2000 Supervision in helping professions, 3rd edn. Open University Press, Oxford

Hawton K 1987 Assessment of suicide risk. British Journal of Psychiatry 150:145–153

Hawton K, Fagg J 1992 Trends in deliberate self-poisoning and self-injury in Oxford, 1976–1990. British Medical Journal 30:1409–1411

Hawton K, Fagg J, McKeown S 1989 Alcoholism, alcohol and attempted suicide. Alcohol and Alcoholism 24(1):3–9

Hawton K, Fagg J, Simkin S et al (unpublished) Attempted suicide in Oxford 1995. University Department of Psychiatry, Warneford Hospital, Oxford

Hawton K, Fagg J, Simkin S, Mills J 1994 The epidemiology of attempted suicide in the Oxford area, England (1989–1992). Crisis 15(3):123–135

Hawton K, van Heeringen C (eds) 2000 The international handbook of suicide and attempted suicide. John Wiley, London

Hawton K, Zahl D, Weatherall R 2003 Suicide following deliberate self-harm: long-term follow-up of patients who present to a general hospital. British Journal of Psychiatry 182:537–542

Health and Welfare Canada 1987 Suicide in Canada: Report of the National Taskforce on Suicide in Canada. Ministry of National Health and Welfare, Ottawa

Health and Welfare Canada 1994 Suicide in Canada: update on the Report of the National Taskforce on Suicide in Canada. Ministry of National Health and Welfare, Ottawa

Heffern WA, Austin W 1999 Compulsory community treatment: ethical considerations. Journal of Psychiatric and Mental Health Nursing 6:37–42

Higgins R, Wistow G, Hurst K 1998 Psychiatric nursing revisited. the care provided for acute psychiatric patients. Whurr, London

Heron J 1990 Helping the client: a creative practical guide. Sage, London

Hill B, Michael S 1996 The human factor. Journal of Psychiatric and Mental Health Nursing 3:245–248

Ho T 2003 The suicide risk of discharged psychiatric patients. Journal of Clinical Psychiatry 64:702–707

Holmes D, Kennedy SL, Perron A 2004 The mentally ill and social exclusion: a critical examination of the use of seclusion from the patient's perspectives. Issues in Mental Health Nursing 25(6):559–578

Hoyer EH, Olesen AV, Mortensen PB 2004 Suicide risk in patients hospitalized because of an affective disorder: a follow-up study, 1973–1993. Journal of Affective Disorders 78:209–217

Humphrey D 1991 Final exit: the practicalities of self-deliverance and assisted suicide for the dying. Hemlock Society, Denver

Hurst K, Wistow G, Higgins R 1999 Mental health nursing in acute settings. Mental Health Practice 4:8–11

Hutchcroft SA, Tanney BL 1989 Sex specific trends in suicide in Canada, 1971–1985. Canadian Journal of Public Health 80:120–123

Hutchinson SA 2000 The development of qualitative health research: taking stock. Qualitative Health Research 11(4):505–521

Issacs S, Keogh S, Menard C, Hockin J 1998 Suicide in the North West Territories: a descriptive review. Chronic Diseases in Canada 19:152–156

Isacsson G, Rich CL 1997 Depression, anti-depressants and suicide: pharmacoepidemiological evidence for suicide prevention In: Maris R et al (eds) Review of suicidology 1997. Guildford Press, New York, p 168–201

Jackson S, Stevenson C 2000 What do people need psychiatric and mental health nurses for? Journal of advanced nursine 31:378–388

Jobes DA, Berman AL 1993 Suicide and malpractice liability: assessing and revising policies, procedures, and practices in out-patient settings. Professional Psychology: Research and Practice 24:91–99

Jobes DA, Luoma JB, Hustead LAT, Mann RE 2000 In the wake of suicide: survivorship and postvention In: Maris RW et al (eds) Comprehensive textbook of suicidology. Guilford Press, New York, p 536–561

Joiner TE 2005 Why people die by suicide. Harvard University Press, Cambridge, MA

Jones J, Jackson A 2004 Observation. In: Harrison M et al (eds) Acute mental health nursing – from acute concerns to the capable practitioner. Sage, London

Jones J, Lowe T, Ward M 2000 Inpatients' experiences of nursing observation on an acute psychiatric unit: a pilot study. Mental Health Care 4:125–129

Jordan JR 2001 Is suicide bereavement different? A reassessment of the literature. Suicide and Life-Threatening Behavior 31(1):91–103

Kant I 1909 Groundwork of the metaphysic of morals. Harper Row, New York

Kato PM, Mann T 1999 A synthesis of psychological interventions for the bereaved (review). Clinical Psychology Review 19(3):275–296

Kavanagh DG 1990 Towards a cognitive-behavioural intervention for adult grief reactions. British Journal of Psychiatry 157:373–383

Keen TM 1999 Schizophrenia: orthodoxy and heresies. A review of alternative possibilities. Journal of Psychiatric and Mental Health Nursing 6:415–424

Kelly S, Charlton J 1995 Suicide deaths in England and Wales, 1982–92: the contribution of occupation and geography. Population Trends 80:16–25

Kerkhof A, Kunst A 1994 A European perspective on suicidal behaviour. In: Jenkins R et al (eds) The prevention of suicide. Department of Health. HMSO, London, p 22–33

Kevorkian J 1991 Prescription medicine: the goodness of planned death. Prometheus Books, New York

Kidd SA 2001 Street youth suicide among an overlooked population Lifenotes 6(1):8–14

Kidd SA, Kral M 2002 Suicide and prostitution among street youth: a qualitative analysis. Adolescene 37: 411–430

King EA, Baldwin DS, Sinclair JMA et al 2001 The Wessex recent in-patient suicide study. 1: case–control study of 234 recently discharged psychiatric patient suicides. British Journal of Psychiatry 178:531–536

Kinmond KS, Bent M 2000 Attendence for self-harm in a west midlands A&E department. British Journal of Nursing 9(4):215–220

Kirmayer LJ 1994 Suicide among Canadian Aboriginal peoples. Transcultural Psychiatric Research Review 31:3–58

Kirmayer L, Boothroyd LJ, Hodgins S 1998 Attempted suicide among Inuit youth: psychosocial correlates and implications for prevention. Canadian Journal of Psychiatry 43:816–822

Kopala B, Kennedy K 1998 Requests for assisted suicide: a nursing issue. Nursing Ethics 5(1):16–26

Krietman N 1977 Parasuicide. Wiley, Chichester

Kvale S 1996 Interviews: an introduction to qualitative research interviewing. Sage, Thousand Oaks

Lavigne-Pley C 1987 Le suicide chez les personnes agees (suicide among the elderly). Canadian Journal of Community Mental Health 6:55–77

Leenaars AA (ed) 1991 Life-span perspectives on suicide: time lines in the suicide process. Plenum, New York

Leenaars A 2004 Psychotherapy with suicidal people: a person-centred approach. John Wiley, Chichester

Leenaars AA, Diekstra R 1997 The will to die: an international perspective. In: Bostis A et al (eds) Suicide: biopsychosocial approaches. Elsevier, Amsterdam, p 241–256

Leenaars AA, Lester D 1994 Domestic and economic correlates of personal violence in Canada and the United States. Italian Journal of Suicidology 4:7–12

Leenaars AA, Lester D 1998 Predicting suicide rates among elderly persons in Canadian provinces. Psychological Reports 82:1202

Leenaars AA, Lester D 1999 Domestic integration and suicide in the provinces of Canada. Crisis 20:59–63

Leenaars AA, Yang B, Lester D 1993 The effects of domestic and economic stress on suicide rates in Canada and the United States. Journal of Clinical Psychology 49:918–921

Leenaars A, De Leo D, Diekstra R et al 1997 Consultations for research in suicidology. Archives of Suicide Research 3:139–151

Lendrum S, Syme G 1992 Gift of tears: a practical approach to loss and bereavement counselling. Routledge, London

Lester D 1988 An analysis of the suicide rate of birth cohorts in Canada. Suicide and Life-Threatening Behavior 18:372–378

Lester D 1992 Why people kill themselves, 3rd edn. CC Thomas, Springfield

Lester D 1995 Suicide in Quebec 1951–1986. Psychological Reports 76:122

Lester D 1996 Suicide rates in Canadian prisons. Perceptual and Motor Skills 81:1230

Lester D 2000 Comparing correlations over time and space. Perceptual and Motor Skills 91:758

Lester D 2002 Qualitative versus quantitative studies in psychiatry: two examples of cooperation from suicidology. Archives of Suicide Research 6(1):15–18

Levy KN, Clarkin JF, Yeomans FE et al 2006 The mechanisms of change in the treatment of borderline personality disorder with transference focused psychotherapy. Journal of Clinical Psychology 62:481–501

Lewis G, Hawton K, Jones P 1997 Strategies for preventing suicide. British Journal of Psychiatry 171:351–354

Libberton P 1996 Depressed and suicidal clients: how nurses can help. Nursing Times 92(43):38–40

Lieberman L 2003 Leaving you: the cultural meanings of suicide. Ivan R Dee, Chicago

Lloyd C 1990 Suicide and self-injury in prison: a literature review. Home Office Research Study No.115. HMSO, London

Lloyd M 1992 Tools for many trades: reaffirming the use of grief counselling by health, welfare and pastoral workers. British Journal of Guidance Counselling 20(2):150–163

Long A, Long A, Smyth A 1998 Suicide: a statement of suffering. Nursing Ethics 5:3–15

Long A, Reid W 1996 An exploration of nurses' attitudes to the nursing care of the suicidal patient in an acute psychiatric ward. Journal of Psychiatric and Mental Health Nursing 3:29–37

McGowan IW, Hamilton S, Miller P, Kernohan G 2005 Contrasting terrorist related deaths with suicide trends over 34 years. Journal of Mental Health 14(4):399–405

McIntosh JL 1993 Control group studies of suicide survivors: a review and critique. Suicide and Life-Threatening Behavior 23:146–160

McIntosh JL 1996 Survivors of suicide: a comprehensive bibliography update, 1986–1995. Omega 33:147–175

McIntyre K, Farrell M, David A 1989 In-patient psychiatric care: the patient's view. British Journal of Medical Psychology 62:249–255

MacKay I, Paterson B, Cassells C 2005 Constant or special observations of inpatients presenting a risk of aggression or violence: nurses' perceptions of the rules of engagement. Journal of Psychiatric and Mental Health Nursing 12(4):464–471

McKenzie I, Wurr C 2001 Early suicide following discharge from a psychiatric hospital. Suicide and Life Threatening Behavior 31:358–363

Maltsberger J 1992 Suicide risk: the formulation of clinical judgement. New York University Press, New York

Maltsberger JT 1998 An explication of rational suicide: its definitions, implications and complications. Journal of Personal and Interpersonal Loss 3:143–159

Maltsbberger JT 2004 Commentary. In: Schneidman E (ed.) Autopsy of a suicidal mind. Oxford University Press, Oxford

Mao Y, Hasselback P, Davies JW et al 1990 Suicide in Canada: an epidemiological assessment. Canadian Journal of Public Health 81(4):324–328

Marcel GG 1948 in Blackham HJ (1986) Six existentialist thinkers. Routledge London, p 140–159

Marion SA, Agbayewa MO, Wiggins S 1999 The effect of season and weather on suicide rates in the elderly in British Columbia. Canadian Journal of Public Health 90:418–422

Maris RW 1981 Pathways to suicide. John Hopkins University Press, Baltimore

Maris RW 1982 Rational suicide. Suicide and Life-threatening Behavior 12(1):3–16

Maris RW 1990 The developmental perspective of suicide. In: Leenaars AA (ed) Life-span perspectives on suicide. Plenum Press, New York

Maris RW 1992 Forensic suicidology. In: Bongar B (ed) Suicide: guidelines for assessment, management and treatment. Oxford University Press, New York, p 235–252

Maris RW 1997a Social forces in suicide: a life review, 1965–1995. In: Maris RW et al (eds) Review of suicidology 1997. Guildford Press, New York, p 42–60

Maris RW 1997b Social suicide. In: Leenaars AA et al (eds) Suicide: individual, cultural, international perspectives. American Association of Suicidology. Guilford Press, New York

Maris RW, Berman AL, Maltsberger JT, Yufit R (eds) 1992 Assessment and prediction of Suicide. Guilford, New York

Maris RW, Berman AL, Silverman MM 2000 Comprehensive textbook of suicidology. Guilford Press, New York

Martocchio BC 1985 Grief and bereavement: healing through hurt. Nursing Clinics of North America 20(2):327–341

Maslow A 1962 Toward a psychology of being. D van Nostrand, Princeton

Meleis AI 1985 Theoretical nursing: development and progress. JB Lippincott, Philadelphia

Mental Health Act (Department of Health 1983) The Mental Health Act. HMSO, London

Mental Health Act Commission and Sainsbury Centre for Mental Health (1997) The National Visit. Sainsbury Centre for Mental Health, London

Mental Health Foundation 2000 Strategies for living. Mental Health Foundation, London

Menzies I 1959/1961 The functioning of social systems as a defence against anxiety: a report on a study of the nursing service of a general hospital. Human Relations 13:95–121

Menzies-Lyth I 1988 Containing anxiety in institutions. Free Association, London

Metz J 2006 Increased risk of lung cancer is not only reason to quit smoking. http://oncolink.com/oncotips/article.cfm?c=s&s=12&ss&id=12

Minois G 2001 History of suicide: voluntary death in Western culture (translated by LG Cochrane). John Hopkins University Press, New York

Mireault D, de Man F 1996 Suicidal ideation among the elderly: personal variables, stress and social support. Social Behaviour and Personality 24:385–392

Mishara BL, Weisstub DN 2005 Ethical and legal issues in suicide research. International Journal of Law and Psychiatry 28:23–41

Moore C 1998 Acute inpatient care could do better, says survey Nursing Times 94(3):54–56

More M 1997 Self-ownership: a core trans-human virtue http://www.maxmore.com/self-own.htm (recovered 2005)

Morgan HG 1994 Assessment of risk. In: Jenkins R et al (eds) The prevention of suicide. HMSO, London, p 49

Morgan HG, Priest P 1991 Suicide and other unexpected deaths among psychiatric in-patients: The Bristol confidential inquiry. British Journal of Psychiatry 158:368–374

Morse JM 1999 Qualitative generalisability. Qualitative Health Research 9(3):5–6

Morse JM, Field PA 1995 Qualitative research methods for health professionals, 2nd edn. Sage, Thousand Oaks

Morttunen M, Aro H, Lonnqvist J 1992 Adolescent suicide: endpoint of long-term difficulties. Journal of the American Academy of Child and Adolescent Psychiatry 31(4):649–654

Moser KA, Goldblatt PO, Fox AJ 1987 Unemployment and mortality: comparison of the 1971 and 1981 longitudinal study census samples. British Medical Journal 294:85–90

Mossey JM, Gallagher RM 2004 The longitudinal occurrence and impact of co-morbid chronic pain and chronic depression over two years in continuing care retirement community residents. Pain Medicine 5(4):335–348

Motto JA 1972 The right to die: a psychiatrist's view. Suicide and Life-Threatening Behavior 2:183–188

Motto JA, Bostrom AG 2001 A randomized controlled trial of postcrisis suicide prevention. Psychiatr Serv 52:828–833

Motto JA, Heilbron DC, Juster RP 1985 Development of a clinical instrument to estimate suicide risk. American Journal of Psychiatry 142:680–686

Munhall P 1982 Nursing philosophy and nursing research: in apposition or opposition? Nursing Research 31(3):176–181

Narveson J 1986 Moral philosophy and suicide. Canadian Journal of Psychiatry 31:104–107

Nasar S 1998 A beautiful mind. Touchstone, New York

Neimeyer RA, Pfeiffer AM 1994 Evaluation of suicide intervention effectiveness. Death Studies 18:131–166

Nolan P 1993 A history of mental health nursing. Chapman & Hall, London

O'Brien AM, Farrell SJ 2005 Community treatment orders: profile of a Canadian experience. Canadian Journal of Psychiatry 50:27–30

O'Reilly RL, Keegan DL, Elias JW 2000 A survey of the use of community treatment orders by psychiatrists in Saskatchewan. Canadian Journal of Psychiatry 45:79–81

Olsen DH, Gorrall DM 2003 Circumplex model of marital and family systems. In: Walsh F (ed.) Normal family process: growing diversity and complexity, 3rd edn. Guildford Press, New York, p 514–548

Orbach I 2003 Suicide and the suicidal body. Suicide and Life-Threatening Behavior 33(1):1–8

Osgood NJ 1991 Psychological factors in late-life suicide. Crisis 12:18–24

Osgood NJ, Brant BA 1990 Suicidal behavior in long-term care facilities. Suicide and Life-Threatening Behavior 20:113–122

Parkes CM 1980 Bereavement counselling: does it work? British Medical Journal 281:3–10

Parkes CM, Brown R 1972 Health after bereavement: a controlled study of young Boston widows and widowers. Psychosomatic Medicine 34:449–461

Pearson A 1992 Knowing nursing: emerging paradigms in nursing. In: Robinson K, Vaughan B (eds) Knowledge for nursing practice. Butterworth Heinemann, Oxford

Peplau H 1952 Interpersonal relations in nursing. Macmillan Press, New York

Peplau H 1988 Interpersonal relations in nursing, 2nd edn. Macmillan Press, New York

Phillips DP, Liu H, Zhang Y 1999 Suicide and social change in China. Culture, Medicine and Psychiatry 22:25–50

Pierce-James I 1967 Suicide and mortality amongst heroin addicts in Britain. British Journal of Addiction 62(3):391–398

Pilgrim D, Rogers A 1999 A sociology of mental health and illness, 2nd edn. Open University Press, Buckingham

Pinhas L, Weaver H, Bryden P et al 2002 Gender role conflict and suicidal behaviour in adolescent girls. Canadian Journal of Psychiatry 47(5):473–476

Plato 1992 Republic (translated by GMA Grube, revised by CDC Reeve). Hackett Publishing Company, Indianapolis

Platt S, Hawton K, Kreitman N et al 1988 Recent clinical and epidemiological trends in para suicide in Edinburgh and Oxford: a tale of two cities. Psychological Medicine 18:405–418

Pokorny AD 1983 Prediction of suicide in psychiatric patients: Report of a prospective study. Archives of General Psychiatry 40:249–257

Pokorny AD 1993 Suicide and prediction revisited. Suicide and Life-threatening Behavior 23:1–10

Popper K 1965 Conjectures and refutations: the growth of scientific knowledge Harper and Row, New York

Powell J, Geddes J, Hawton K 2000 Suicide in psychiatric hospital in-patients. British Journal of Psychiatry 176(3):266–272

Prado CG 1998 The last chance, pre-emptive suicide in old age. Prager, West Point

Prigerson HG, Frank E, Kasl SV et al 1995 Complicated grief and bereavement-related depression as distinct disorders: Preliminary empirical validation in elderly bereaved spouses. American Journal of Psychiatry 152(1):22–30

Pritchard C 1993 Psychosocioeconomic factors in suicide. Cited in Thompson T, Rawlins RP (1993) Hope-hopelessness. In: Rawlins RP et al (eds) Mental health-psychiatric nursing: a holistic life-cycle approach. Mosby, St Louis MO

Pritchard C 1998 Psychosocialeconomic factors in suicide. In: Thompson T, Matthias P (eds) Lyttle's Mental Health and Disorder, 2nd edn. Bailliere Tindall, London, p 276–295

Qin P, Nordentoft M 2005 Suicide risk in relation to psychiatric hospitalization. Evidence based on longitudinal registers. Archives of General Psychiatry 62:427–432

Quan H, Arboleda-Florez J, Fich CH et al 2002 Association between physical illness and suicide among the elderly. Social Psychiatry and Psychiatric Epidemiology 37:190–197

Ramcharan P, Cutcliffe JR 2001 Judging the ethics of qualitative research: considering the 'ethics' as process model. Health and Social Care 9(6):358–367

Ranieri WF, Steer RA, Lavrence TI et al 1987 Relationship of depression, hopelessness and dysfunctional attitudes to suicide in psychiatric patients. Psychological Reports 61:967–975

Raphael B, Middleton W 1987 Current state of research in the field of bereavement. Israel Journal of Psychiatry and Related Sciences 24(1–2):5–32

Raphael B, Middleton W, Martinek N et al 1993 Counselling and therapy of the bereaved. In: Stroebe M et al (eds) Handbook of bereavement: theory, research and intervention. Cambridge University Press, New York

Rawlins RP 1993 Hope-hopelessness. In: Rawlins et al (eds) Mental health nursing – a holistic life cycle approach, 3rd edn. Mosby, St Louis, p 257–284

Reed J, Camus J, Last JM 1985 Suicide in Canada:birth cohort analysis. Canadian Journal of Public Health 38:9–14

Reynolds D 2006 House of Lords soundly rejects assisted suicide proposal. http://raggedmagazine.com/ide/assisted_suicide/00141.html

Rich AR, Bonner RL 1987 Concurrent validity of a stress-vulnerability model of suicidal ideation and behavior: a follow up study. Suicide and Life-Threatening Behavior 17:265–270

Rich AR, Kirkpatrick-Smith J, Bonner RL, Jans F 1992 Gender differences in the psycho-social correlates of suicide ideation among adolescents. Suicide and Life-Threatening Behavior 22:364–373

Ritter S 1989 Manual of clinical psychiatric nursing and procedures. Harper Row, London

Robinson J, Meehan J, Appleby L 2002 Safety first recommendations from the five-year report of the National Confidential Inquiry into suicide and homicide by people with mental illness. NHSLA Review, issue 23

Rogers A, Pilgrim D 2001 Mental health policy in Britain: a critical introduction, 2nd edn. Macmillan, Basingstoke

Rogers A, Pilgrim D, Lacey R 1993 Experiencing psychiatry: users' views of services Macmillan/MIND, London

Roy A 1982 Risk factors for suicide in psychiatric patients. Archives of General Psychiatry 39:1089–1095

Rudd DM 2000 Integrating science into the practice of clinical suicidology: a review of the psychotherapy literature and a research agenda for the future. In: Maris RW et al (eds) Review of suicidology. Guildford Press, New York, p 47–86

Rudman MJ 1996 User involvement in the nursing curriculum: seeking users' views. Journal of Psychiatric and Mental Health Nursing 3:195–200

Rutz W, Carlsson P, von Knorring L, Walinder J 1992a Cost-benefit analysis of an educational program for general practitioners by the Swedish Committee for the Prevention and Treatment of Depression. Acta Psychiatrica Scandinavica 85(6):457–464

Rutz W, von Knorring L, Walinder J 1992b Long-term effects of an educational program for general practitioners given by the Swedish Committee for the Prevention and Treatment of Depression. Acta Psychiatrica Scandinavica 85(1):83–88

Rutz W, Walinder J, Eberhard G et al. 1989 An educational program on depressive disorders for general practitioners on Gotland: background and evaluation. Acta Psychiatrica Scandinavica 79(1):19–26

Samuelsson M, Wiklander M, Asberg M, Saveman B 2000 Psychiatric are as seen by the attempted suicide patient. Journal of Advanced Nursing 2:635–643

Sandelowski M 1997 'To be of use': enhancing the utility of qualitative research. Nursing Outlook 45(3):125–132

Sanon-Rollins G Surviving conflict on the job nursing spectrum: students corner (recovered 2006) http://www.nursingspectrum.com/StudentsCorner/StudentFeatures/Surviving Conflict_stk04.htm

Santa Mina EE, Gallop R 1998 Childhood sexual and physical abuse and adult self-harm and suicidal behaviour: a literature review. Canadian Journal of Psychiatry 43(8): 793–800

Satre JP 1943 In: Blackham HJ (1986) Six existentialist thinkers. Routledge London, p 58–79

Schneider J 1985 Hopelessness and helplessness. Journal of Psychosocial Nursing and Mental Health Services 23:12–21

Schofield P 2005 Effects of chronic pain: In: Schofield P (ed) Beyond pain. Whurr, London

Schotte DE, Clum G 1987 Problem-solving skills in suicidal psychiatric patients. Journal of Consulting and Clinical Psychology 55(1):49–54

Schut HAW, Stroebe MS, Van den Bout J et al 1997 Intervention for the bereaved: gender differences in the efficacy of two counselling programmes. British Journal of Clinical Psychology 36:63–72

Scottish Executive 2002 Choose life: a national strategy and action plan to prevent suicide in Scotland. Scottish Executive, Edinburgh

Scruby LS, Sloan JA 1989 Evaluation of bereavement interventions. Canadian Journal of Public Health 80:394–398

Shneidman ES 1972 Foreward. In: Cain AC (ed) Survivors of suicide (p ix–xi). Charles C Thomas, Springfield IL

Shneidman ES 1973 Suicide. In: Encyclopedia Britannica, 21:383–385, Williams Benton, Chicago

Shneidman ES 1985 Definition of suicide. John Wiley, New York

Shneidman ES 1997 The suicidal mind. In: Maris RW et al (eds) Review of suicidology. Guildford Press, New York, p 22–41

Shneidman ES 2004 Autopsy of a suicidal mind. Oxford University Press, Oxford

Sigurdson E, Staley D, Matas M et al 1994 A five year review of youth suicide in Manitoba. Canadian Journal of Psychiatry 39(8):397–403

Silverman MM 1997 Current controversies in suicidology. In: Maris RW et al (eds) Review of suicidology. Guildford Press, New York, p 1–21

Silverman MM 2000 Rational suicide, hastened death and self-destructive behaviours. The Counselling Psychologist 28:445–510

Slaby AE 1994 Pharmacotherapy of suicide. In: Leenaars AA et al (eds) Treatment of suicidal people. Taylor Francis, New York

Sloan N, Leon-Camacho WL, Rojas PE et al 1994 Kangaroo mother method: randomized control trial of an alternative method of care for stabilizing low birth weight infants. Lancet 344:782–785

Smith K, Biley F 1997 Understanding grounded theory: principles and evaluation. Nurse Researcher 4(3):17–30

Speijer N, Diekstra R 1980 Assisted suicide: a study of the problems related to self chosen death. Preventer, van Loughun Slaterur

Standing Nursing and Midwifery Advisory Committee 1999 Practice guidance: safe and supportive observation of patients at risk: mental health nursing – addressing acute concerns. Department of Health, London

Stevenson C 2005 Postmodern clinical supervision in nursing. Issues in Mental Health Nursing 26(5):519–530

Stevenson C, Cutcliffe J 2006 Using Foucault to analyse special observations in psychiatry: genealogy, discourse and power/knowledge. Journal of Psychiatric and Mental Health Nursing 13:713–721

Strachan J, Johansen H, Nair C, Nargundkar M 1990 Canadian suicide mortality rates: first generation immigrants versus Canadia-born. Health Reports 2:327–341

Stravynski A, Boyer R 2001 Loneliness in relation to suicide ideation and parasuicide: a population-wide study. Suicide and Life-Threatening Behavior 31(1):32–40

Stuart GW 2001 Self-protective responses and suicide. In: Stuart GW, Laria MT (eds) Principles and practices of psychiatric nursing, 7th edn. Mosby, New York, p 381–401

Stuart CW, Sundine SJ 1991 Principles and practice of psychiatric nursing. Mosby, Toronto

Sun FK, Long A, Boore J, Tsao LI 2005 Nursing people who are suicidal on psychiatric wards in Taiwan: action and interaction strategies. Journal of Psychiatric and Mental Health Nursing 12(3):275–282

Surg HB 2006 Health risks of obesity. http://www.annecollins.com/obesity/risks-of-obesity.htm

Szasz T 1985 Suicide: what is the physician's responsibility? Unpublished paper presented at the Harvard Medical School

Szasz T 1990 The untamed tongue. Open Court Publishing, Chicago

Takahashi Y 1997 Culture and suicide from a Japanese psychiatrist's perspective. In Leenaars AA, Maris RW, Takahashi Y (eds) Suicide: Individual, cultural and international perspectives. Guildford, New York p 137–145

Talseth AG, Lindseth A, Jacobson L, Norberg A 1997 Nurses' narrations about suicidal psychiatric inpatients. Nord Jour Psychiatry 51:359–364

Talseth AG, Lindseth A, Jacobson L, Norberg A 1999 The meaning of suicidal in-patients' experiences of being cared for by mental health nurses. Journal of Advanced Nursing 29(5):1034–1041

Tanney BL 2000 Psychiatric diagnoses and suicidal acts. In: Maris RW et al (eds) Comprehensive textbook of suicidology. Guildford Press, New York, p 311–340

Task Force on Suicide in Canada 1994 Suicide in Canada: update of the Report of The Task Force of Suicide in Canada. Mental Health Division – Health Services Directorate, Health Programs and Services Branch, Canada

Tatai K 1991 Suicide in the elderly: a report from Japan. Crisis 12:40–43

Ten Have HAMJ, Weile JVM, Spicer SF 1998 Ownership of the human body: philosophical considerations on the use of human body and its parts in health care. Kluwer, New York

Tesch RS, Denardin OVP, Baptista CA, Dias FL 2004 Depression levels in chronic orofacial pain patients: a pilot study. Journal of Oral Rehabilitation 31:926–932

Torre E, Chieppa N, Freilone F 1988 Gestes suicidaires et solitude (suicidal behavior loneliness). Psychologie Medicale 20:342–344

Trout DL 1980 The role of social isolation in suicide. Suicide and Life-threatening Behavior 10(1):10–23

Trovato F 1986 Suicide and ethnic factors in Canada. International Journal of Social Psychiatry 32:55–64

Trovato F 1991 Sex, marital status and suicide in Canada. Sociological Perspectives 34:427–445

Tschudin V 1997 Counselling for loss and bereavement Bailliere Tindall, London

Turk DC, Okifuji A, Scharff L 1995 Chronic pain and depression: role of perceived impact and perceived control in different age groups. Pain 61:93–101

Van Der Wal J 1989 The aftermath of suicide: a review of the empirical evidence. Omega 20:149–171

Van Pragg HM 2004 Stress and suicide – are we well equipped to study this issue? Crisis 25(2):80–85

Walen S 2002 It's a funny thing about suicide: a personal experience. British Journal of Guidance Counselling 30:415–430

War Resisters International Council 2005 Statement by the War Resisters' International Council, Seoul, South Korea, July 2nd, 2005
http://www.wri-irg.org/statemnt/finland05council-en.htm

Ward MW, Jones J 2006 Close observations: the scapegoat of mental health care? In: Cutcliffe JR, Ward MW (eds) Key debates in psychiatric/mental health care nursing. Elsevier, Edinburgh, p 242–256

Weishaar ME 2000 Cognitive risk factors in suicide. In: Maris R et al (eds) Review of suicidology. Guilford Press, New York, p 112–139

Welu T 1977 A follow-up program for suicide attempters: evaluation of effectiveness. Suicide and Life-threatening Behavior 7:17–30

Wenz FV 1977 Marital status, anomie, and forms of social isolation: a case of high suicide rate among the widowed in an urban sub-area. Diseases of the Nervous System 38(11): 891–895

Werth JL 1996 Rational suicide? Implications for mental health professionals. Brunner/Mazel, Philadelphia

Werth JL (ed) 1999 Contemporary perspectives on rational suicide. Brunner/Mazel, Philadelphia

White J 2003 Report on the workshop on suicide-related research in Canada. Canadian Institutes of Health Research/Health Canada, Ottawa

Wise T 2003 Waking up: climbing through the darkness. Pathfinder, Oxnard, California

Worden JW 1988 Grief counselling and grief therapy. Tavistock/Routledge, London

World Health Organization 2002 Website address www.int/health_topics/suicide/en/

World Health Organization 2005 The Regional Director for the Western Pacific, WHO, Suicide Prevention in the Western Pacific Region website address www.who.int/regional_director/speeches

Young MA, Fogg LF, Schefter WA, Fawcett JA 1994 Interactions of risk factors in predicting suicide. American Journal of Psychiatry 151(3):434–435

LAW REFERENCES

Bolam versus Frien Hospital Management Committee (1957) 2 All ER 118, (1957) 1 WLR 582

R versus Adams (1957) Crim. LR 365

R versus Cox (1992) 12 BMLR 38

Airedale NHS Trust v Bland (1993) 1 All ER 821

http://www.survivorsofsuicide.com/beyond_surviving.shtml

Index